Wise Secrets of Aloha

Learn and Live the
Sacred Art of Lomilomi

Kahuna Harry Uhane Jim
and Garnette Arledge

WEISER BOOKS
San Francisco, CA / Newburyport, MA

First published in 2007 by Weiser Books
an imprint of Red Wheel/Weiser, LLC
With offices at:
500 Third Street, Suite 230
San Francisco, CA 94107
www.redwheelweiser.com

ISBN-10: 1-57863-398-2
ISBN-13: 978-1-57863-398-2

Library of Congress Cataloging-in-Publication Data

Jim, Harry Uhane.
Wise secrets of aloha : learn and live the sacred art
of lomilomi / Harry Uhane Jim and Garnette Arledge.
p. cm.
ISBN 1-57863-398-2 (alk. paper)
1. Spiritual healing--Hawaii. 2. Hawaii--Religion. 3. Massage--Hawaii.
4. Kahuna. I. Arledge, Garnette. II. Title.
BL2620.H3J56 2007
299'.9242--dc22   2006033873

Cover and text design by Kathryn Sky-Peck
Typeset in Sabon
Cover photograph © Corbis Images
TCP
10 9 8 7 6 5 4 3 2 1

To the *Halau Uhane Lomilomi Lapaʻau*
With grand joy in rainbow colors, my dedication celebrates
my wife, Sila's, profound and radiant love in my life and
those of our children, Leinani, Kalaʻe, Kapono, Keani, and Keola.
Aloha Nui Nui to Sila Lehua.
—KAHUNA HARRY UHANE JIM

To my children, Elizabeth and Drew, and his children,
Lilly and Alex, with great love.
To Christopher Stickler, who believes in my work
and knows the truth within these pages.
—GARNETTE ARLEDGE

Contents

Preface

Our great and glorious masterpiece is to live appropriately....
The most certain sign of wisdom is cheerfulness.
—Michel de Montaigne

Aloha calls. Listen into the breeze, the splash of waves—the air is filled with Aloha. Listen, you are being called to the Aloha Spirit in the book you are holding. Listen as I did. All the abundance, freedom from cherished wounds, and joy you have ever yearned for can be yours with the Aloha Spirit. I know, for Aloha called me at just the right time. Aloha can change your life as it did mine.

For a lifetime spent writing articles and books, I've also spent thirty years doing energy work and hands-on healing. Working with death, the dying, and hospices grew out of my experiences of profound love and provided an opportunity for service to those who suffer. If pressed, I might say I am a practicing mystic, but I'd rather say I'm a regular person. I have dedicated my adult life to honoring and studying the Divine One, whose breath impinges upon world religions as many names. I love the deep life. Perhaps that's why I got into hospice work, first as a trainer of volunteers and then as a chaplain. I wrote a book called *On Angel's Eve* for family members because I longed to help people overcome their fear of dying.

Then suddenly my partner, cocreator of our golden quest, was killed on the New York Thruway while he was changing a tire. Everything changed.

Let's skip the grimy details of my own grief process and get right back to the state of mind called Hawaii. Once the *Angel's* book was finished, I began praying for another life affirming, deeply spiritual topic to write about next. While I was still carrying the burden of missing my partner so terribly, I was invited to cook for a multiday Hawaiian workshop. So I laughed and said yes, because cooking in a way is like writing. Bringing beautiful colors and fresh organic nourishment to bless and enliven others— that's a book as well as a meal. The workshop was being given by an authentic native Hawaiian kahuna, and his teaching was on Lomilomi, the delicious healing-touch therapy of the Islands. Lomilomi's primary definition, one of its many definitions, is to raise the vibration of the receiver. That's what I am married to as a theology, to raise vibrations, for goodness sake. Here's the picture: it's the western Catskills, not too near Oneonta, New York. I'm cooking in the school's brand new kitchen. Up drives a Dodge Caravan, and from the backseat emerges the six-foot Hawaiian kahuna with his curly black hair, bare feet, and shorts (it's early April in upstate New York, there's still snow on the ground, and he's in shorts). He is laughing. He has a very large presence. That's how I first met Harry Uhane Jim.

Having felt the vibration of cooking chaos miles away, he puts on his sandals, mushes across the snowy yard, saunters into the steamy kitchen, offering at once—right after a six-hour car trip— to help prep the food. Rising to help, even in the kitchen, now that's a true healer. His first assignment: wrestle open a dozen spaghetti squash. With his massive hands, he takes the knife, and in one swift cut each opens. For Harry, who uses gravity and a giggle, it seems like cutting pie. Then he invites me to join the workshop, which I do during cooking breaks. And during their workshop breaks, he and his wife join me in the kitchen to help out.

Here's another picture: During the workshop, a friend and I are learning about the Creating Space technique. The first time I am a receiver on the table. I lie there with my eyes closed, trusting the process. Harry walks over, sticks his great hand into my heart chakra, that area from the top of the spiritual heart to just under the ribcage and above the diaphragm. In a flash I release a great big bag of mourning. In a second, literally, the grief flies out. I feel wave after wave of release. Rushes of energy pour through my heart and out the top of my head, then I feel an enormous, cosmos-size gratitude and brilliance. It is a huge Gratitude Wave. All I can do is laugh, grin, and smile with gratitude. Then Harry's wife of twenty-five years, Sila (pronounced with a long i, as in "silo") holds my feet to ground me back on the planet. I find myself again. That's vintage Harry.

One final picture: During the last treatment of the workshop, when my colleague Sue Ann Wilkerson is the giver, an enormous healing guardian seems to stand stalwart over the massage table where I lie soaking in the Aloha and says to me: "Write a book about Aloha and Lomilomi."

Synchronistically, Harry comes over as this vision is happening, so I put the suggestion to him.

One month later, after pondering, he said no. Later, I asked again; he said no. I asked a third time, as I really, really felt guided to do this; he laughed. Hawaiians know you have to ask three times. He was not playing three questions games with me. He was really, really reluctant to do it until his guidance confirmed that it was time.

The reluctant teacher, he did not want to lift the orchid curtain or set himself up in aggrandizement. Kahunas are keepers of the deep mysteries, steeped in the oral tradition, which is transmitted lineage to lineage, person by person. But the book was not in either of our hands alone—the Halau guardians know that the Whole Earth needs these gentle teachings now.

When Harry finally agreed, we were sitting on a balcony back at the school in the western Catskills. At the very moment he said yes, a bald eagle flew overhead. Later, as we were driving, he stopped the van suddenly. We watched a turtle the size of a Thanksgiving platter cross the road. "That's the blessing," Harry said.

We considered deeply before committing to this work. If someone authentic and Hawaiian does not teach them, these healings will disappear from the planet with the passing of Harry Uhane Jim, the last kahuna of Lomilomi. Then our publisher, Weiser Books, for the past fifty years one of the most respected names for deep esoteric and metaphysical books, stepped forward. I knew then that the Halau guardians were leading this concert.

We got to work, and so, here it is, *Wise Secrets of Aloha*. Enjoy. Laugh a lot. Be easygoing. Go easy. Listen to the air. There's an inner island paradise waiting for you in these pages ahead.

—REV. GARNETTE ARLEDGE, M.DIV.
St. Hilda's Lodge, Woodstock, New York

Calling the Wave

Ho'opiapia O Ke Nalu
Now! *Ho*, dear reader, call the wave to you so you may be in the *Pa'a*, the
now, as you read, understand, and become one with the legendary
Hawaiian islands that are called truly paradise. *Ho'opaipai*. Aloha!
—Kahuna Harry Uhane Jim

Let's start easy. We really want you to move the energy in your
body into harmony, happiness, and gratitude. So here's your
flight ticket—you are welcome with Aloha to enter the realm of
the Hawaiian Temple Lomilomi with kahuna Harry Uhane Jim,
initiated priest of the traditional mysteries of Hawaii. What is a
kahuna? Why enter the *Halau* space? And what is the Temple
Lomilomi? Your questions will be answered as the waves of understanding flow in.

In this book you will learn the sacred flow of Hawaiian words,
words carrying healing, mystery, beauty, and spiritual depth. Words
have power. Let's start with the traditional chant of the legendary
surfers: *Ho'opaipai O Ke Nalu*—call the wave. It is both a surrender
to the mighty ocean and a command flying gloriously over it, calling
in the perfect wave for surfing, *Ho'opaipai O Ke Nalu*—show up
perfect wave, please. So I can meet you. So I can be receiving.

In the early twentieth century, schoolteacher Max Freedom Long spent two decades searching fruitlessly, both in Hawaii and in the United States for the key to unpacking the language of the Hawaiian oral esoteric tradition. Then he awoke in the middle of the night with the sudden inspiration that the Hawaiian language is actually a code. In a synchronistic moment, thanks to the dream-gift of the kahunas, Long decoded some of the ancient language used by the kahunas to describe their wisdom teachings. But not all, much was still hidden.

What he missed was that Hawaiian is a *vibrational* code. Actually, Hawaiian is a language of vibrations and feelings. And the predominant emotion is Aloha. Long did not know then that he had found the tip of a complex healing system able to synthesize Freudian terms for unconscious and conscious states and neurolinguistics. At that time, Freudian psychoanalytical terms and linguistic analysis of words were in their infancy; both were new to Western concepts, but not to Hawaiian kahunas.

From a sudden waking, Long went on, painstakingly, following the string bit by bit, to turn the golden key to the carefully locked kahuna ways. He was then able to discover only a few of the psychic principles kahunas use for healing. Long never was able to make contact with any native Hawaiian healers, but perhaps his dedication and purity of intention, his light, attracted the Halau guardians, who gave him access to the threshold. It is up to the seeker to come to the threshold, but only the Spirit carries the seeker inside.

Pay attention—*Ho*—then, in this book to the sacred language of Hawaii, as Harry Uhane Jim unpacks the healing ways of Lomilomi for you. This book is your golden key to the paradise that is Hawaiian, and that is universal.

In an ideal world, it is best to learn Hawaiian shamanism and its ways from, of course, a born Hawaiian. But that's complicated in the twenty-first century. Two hundred years of pleasure seekers, whether the pleasure is trade, religion, or fun, have diluted access to the old ways. However, wisdom from its own members is vital to understanding a metaphysical, earth-based spiritual tradition. Before outsiders can interpret them, spiritual traditions must be given in the first-person voice.

What Is a Kahuna to Hawaiians?

So to answer the question "what is a kahuna?" let's start by declaring that a kahuna is only someone who has, by lineage of blood, birth, and initiation, become so deeply interwoven with the teachings that there is no difference between the teaching and the teacher. The wisdom is fully integrated in the exemplary life and body of the kahuna.

Kahuna, according to kahuna Papa David Kaonohiokala Bray, the grandfather of Harry's wife Sila, is a compound word from *kahu*, meaning an honored or high servant/caretaker who has or takes charge of persons or property, and *na*, meaning calmness and quiet evolution of the emotions. Thus, a kahuna is the calm, high servant of those who may be seeking higher emotional evolution. In other words, like all real leaders and healers, a kahuna serves the community. You see how this definition goes further into what *kahuna* means than the definition used by researcher Long, who said *Ka* means "the" and *huna* means "concealed knowledge." Long's "concealed knowledge" is quite a distance in meaning from "keeper of the secrets" in Hawaiian. Harry defines *kahuna* as "a keeper of the wise and hidden secrets." *Ka* is also the root syllable of *Kane*, the Hawaiian triune "being of humanness." *Kane,* whose vibratory meaning, according to Harry, is the congress of our three selves. Papa Bray taught that kahunas are a class of trained people who serve humanity for goodness and truth. When kahunas are trained, they are anchored in knowing God in all life. Kahunas align to the God of Light within.

For ages, kahunas were the powers of the Hawaiian monarchy. Kahunas specialized; some were prime ministers and judges, others heads of sacred space (church) or the sacramental *hula* dance, and some the doctors or healers to their people. Some were sorcerers rather than healers (see chapter 7).

What Is the Halau?

In order to understand deeply the esoteric and gracious Hawaiian ways, one must approach with respect, withholding judgment through humility, and listen clearly. For as you read, you automatically enter into the *Halau*, the esoteric field of the Temple Lomilomi, traditional Hawaiian healing-touch medicine (see chapter 2). The Halau can be defined as the continuum's comfort zone where we can learn. The Halau is all forces for good gathering to help us learn. The Halau guardians are multidimensional beings who support healing. When you enter the Halau, elders or guardians on the esoteric plane gather to meet you on this plane.

Intertwined like the maile vine around the painted eucalyptus tree in the Wainiha rainforest are the spirituality and the healing methods of traditional Hawaii. Spirituality and healing are one to the native Hawaiians. The religious well-being of the isles is to the Hawaiian priest-kahuna all about healing—physical, mental, emotional, and therefore spiritual healing, all at the same time. For example, the hula dancers, says Harry, are heart-sweet souls dedicated to the dance art form. Doing the hula, you experience the same sweet warmth as being in the Halau. Sila, Harry's wife of twenty-five years and mother of their five children, is a hula *kumu*, a teacher of the sacred dance.

Thus entering the Halau (the esoteric field for creating knowledge) is about expanding skills, empowering accuracy, and abundantly manifesting the healing ability by engaging with emotions. Persons ill in body would come to the kahunas for total wellness. We now call that holistic healing. In old Hawaii, it was the traditional, orthodox path of medicine—and to many, still is. Whether the problem was relationships, work, childbearing, dying, possession, psychological or mental wounds, physical manifestations of those emotional disruptions, or addictions, the people came to their neighbors and family who had been trained from earliest years to take care of their needs.

Why Were the Kahuna Hidden?

It seems the various missionaries and immigrants rang a death toll for the population of 300,000 island-born Hawaiians. After healers were outlawed in the 1870s, fewer than 60,000 survived. *Genocide* is the modern term for what continues to happen to Hawaiian people. Not only did the newcomers bring diseases unsuited to the immune systems of the native people, but they also ignorantly outlawed the very persons who could have treated those diseases.

So, like the wisdom of other invaded peoples, the healing wisdom of the Hawaiians went into hiding and the healers went behind a curtain—in this case an orchid curtain. The community knew their healers and leaders, but it was vital that the newcomers, the *ha'ole* did not. (*Ha* means " breath," *ole* means "no," therefore "a person with no breath showing.") Prison and death would result if the healers were known, so they quietly kept close to *Aina*, the land, hidden but in plain view. Traditional priests were affectionately camouflaged, as the words *uncle* or *auntie* or *Papa* or *Daddy* masked the revered title of *kahuna*. The rule of denial, the attitude of "don't know anything," was prevalent, hiding the healing truths behind a hospitable exterior, yet giving no real healing information away to the curious.

Secret initiations continued, as the old ones recognized from within those who had been born to carry on the teachings. The elders could recognize those who had the powerful inner destiny to be kahunas. These new healers were gathered, adopted, and initiated into the kahuna tradition, all with just a look that was perhaps only two to three seconds long.

Assimilation and survival for the Hawaiians has meant intermarriage with the Asian (Japanese, Filipino, Chinese, Korean) and European (German, Portuguese, Norwegian, Irish, American) seekers of paradise. People with one half Hawaiian ancestry are considered legally Hawaiian and able to own traditional lands. Now, shockingly, there are only seven or eight thousand people of full Hawaiian blood still living. Mind and heart boggling as this is, this is what has happened in the beloved islands. It was only the passing of the Religious Freedom Act of 1978 (Public Law 95-341) that freed the kahuna from their rainforest shadows.

What Is the Temple Lomilomi?

The Temple Lomilomi is the rest of the book. On a menu, *Lomilomi* means a dish of delicious red salmon fresh from the ocean with raw red onions, salad dressing, and Hawaiian spices and herbs. On a different level, *Lomilomi* means touch-therapy body work. *Lomi* means "energy shift" and "thumb." *Lomilomi* means energy-shifting touch therapy that can change your mind, body, emotions, and life for the good. There are different versions of Lomilomi— some gentle, some quick and commercial, some deep and intense. In Lomilomi, what would be called the practitioner in other modalities is called the giver. The client is called the receiver. Giver and receiver are gentler, less hierarchical terms. Healers know that the one on the table gives as well as receives, and vice versa.

But the word has a more fundamental meaning. *Lomi* means, in the Hawaiian language, to take and turn, to shift. When Hawaiians say a word twice, they are emphasizing the weight of importance, hence: Lomilomi. When we speak of the art of Lomilomi here, we are speaking of the sacred shift within you that is inspired by the healing kahuna raising your vibration and all that is around you.

Lomilomi comes from the *Aina*, meaning land. The Aina holds the wise secrets of Hawaii in her safekeeping. The very land is sacred and so are the beings that live with her in harmony. Now, because of the diminished population and increased world dishar-mony, the Halau elders, guardians, and ancestors are pressing for the secret teaching to be brought to light in an undistorted way by one of their own, kahuna Harry Uhane Jim. In these pages, Kahuna Harry will introduce you to the Lomilomi way of life.

So, come to the islands with us. You are invited with all the hospitality of Aloha to come in. Welcoming, saying "Ho'opaipai O Ke Nalu," we encircle you with Aloha blessings. May you feast on the concepts of Lomilomi. May you too become an adept at Lomilomi. May the Breath of God, the One Source that is in our presence, be generous to you as you experience the Temple Lomilomi in this book.

Part One

Calling and Feeding
the Aloha Spirit

IN PART ONE WE WILL DIVE into the sacred levels of Hawaiian teachings: language, blessing, the Aloha spirit, and the three selves within each individual person. Supporting each chapter are healing stories, usually told in Harry's first-person voice, but sometimes by his receivers.

Wise Secrets of Aloha begins with the presence of God's breath. Please take a deep cleansing breath now.

Aloha is about the deep mysteries of the Hawaiian kahunas. Through these pages you will ineffably experience the Temple Lomilomi. Temple Lomilomi healing work transforms the person into an actual temple in which time, space, and will converge for physical and emotional healing and for a life of fun, abundance, and laughter. Hawaii's traditional Lomilomi approach sings with joy, blessing, and healing. We're going to have fun expanding the light of Lomilomi healing.

In chapter one we will look at the Hawaiian concept of vertical time, which is so very different from linear "clock" time, Harry's kahuna lineage, and *Iʻo*, the hawk. Then you will learn how to slip from one dimension to another, from time to no-time, from linear time to vertical time and back, from past, present, and future to *Paʻa*, the now. All of these dimensions are part of what Aloha means on the more subtle levels.

Chapter two is dedicated to deepening the visceral understanding of the essence of Aloha. Unpack each syllable by shaking the sand out of your beach sandals and any preconceived notions you have of Aloha.

Chapter three brings you into the Temple Lomilomi. The first Lomilomi technique is Creating Space. There is outer, interstellar space and inner, personal space. Harry introduces the Hawaiian connection with the Pleiades Beings of Light and the inner connection with your own light center of gratitude. Once you have a handle on the basic Aloha terms, you can expect the activation of the Gratitude Point that lives within each and every one of us.

It all begins with Aloha. Let the Aloha Spirit wrap you in welcome and healing as Harry shares the intimate knowledge of the meaning of Hawaii's sacred language of rounded vowels and happy endings. Aloha!

Preparing the Path

O Great Spirit, please open the path on which we travel.
You go before us; you go behind us,
On the right, on the left, above and below us.
If we should err, in thoughts, in deeds,
Or in treading of our feet, be compassionate with us.
Be our guide. It is finished. It is free.

CHAPTER ONE

The Esoteric Aloha Spirit

A Ke Akua! By your power and agreement,
I declare: Open the Port.
—ancient Hawaiian invocation

Welcome to Hawaii, where every leaf, every rock, every person, every waterfall, the waves, the ocean, the beach, the scented trade winds, and all life is a manifestation of divine energy and brimming with Aloha for you.

In this place, this space, the reigning idea is that, as God sees us, no one is above the other. So humans see God in every form, and in no form there is not God's presence. Hawaii's secret of paradise is Aloha: "the breath of God is in our presence."

Aloha, the beloved greeting for hello and good-bye known the world over, is a many-leveled, truly multisplendored healing sound all by itself. There is in all creation, in Aloha, a bigger, wider, more substantive presence of spirituality than we can, at the surface, see or know.

So say Aloha now to yourself. Savor Aloha, the traditional greeting. Generosity offers you a scented white-ginger lei. You are the welcomed guest. Aloha overflows with hospitality, flashes abundance, and offers beauty to all.

Thus, each person honored with Aloha feels loved, feels welcomed, feels beauty, feels warmth, and therefore feels joy. Emotions swim with delight; healing occurs. The separation of strangers is replaced with the natural warmth of being loved, being supported. When the plane touches down in Honolulu, the tradition is that beauties rush forward gracefully, singing Aloha, and placing leis around the necks of newcomers.

More spirituality is going on here than is apparent to the physical eyes. This Aloha welcoming ritual is designed to raise the vibration of the travel-weary newcomer to these islands that are the most remote from any of the continents on Earth. Aloha calls forth, soul to soul, the spirit of generosity and hospitality. In knowingly greeting newcomers with Aloha, invoking the presence of God within, automatically, the vibrations of the travel-weary visitor are raised, thus benefiting all. Harry calls this process vivification—revving up the energy, raising good spiritual feelings. Is this a working definition of Hawaiian theology? Yes, partially, according to the Halau Uhane Lomilomi Lapa'au, Harry and Sila's esoteric school for creating knowledge of the spirit of healing-touch medicine.

Harry says healing is the inalienable inheritance of each human. Healing transforms the person into an actual temple in which time, space, and will converge. Each person is a temple. Then, knowing of such healing, each person can say, "Lomilomi is a commitment to myself. My presence here is a sacred manifestation from me to myself to shower gratitude, growth, and bliss to my whole being. I focus to enter into and sustain my temple in the heart, the *pu'u*."

Swimming into the depths of knowledge requires healing of the cherished wounds and tantrums of the past, present, and future, all lurking within the body-mind-emotional system of an individual.

You become the temple so that energy moves from the heart, and through the heart moves the essence of your own light, your *Uhane* (see chapter two), your support, guide, and grace. You will begin each Lomilomi session with a receiver's opportunity to commit to the experience by saying these words:

I commit the energy of certainty to the abundance and perfection of my intuition, as I am radiant in the light of Aloha.

Make this your own pledge.

So let us begin with the teaching. First: the symbol of Thundering Grace. (See illustration on page 7.)

This complex symbol pictures both God's grace and human's gratitude back to God. Not the God of our understanding, but to Hawaiian kahunas, God grander than our ability to hold in the mind. Light is another Hawaiian code word for God. Light is defined as having a conscious connection to God. Light that feeds the human's call for grace by sending Spirit, which regenerates and strengthens humans. That grace is inalienable and freely given. That grace is the unmerited favor and love of God. In turn, we feed the Light through gratitude, or the state of being grateful. The symbol pictures God's reaction to our call. This crosscurrent of energy generates grace receiving gratitude.

OPPORTUNITY

Be comfortable. Adjust and trust yourself. Fill yourself with gratitude and bliss. This is an opportunity to emotionally invest in your Higher Self. When you breathe three full relaxing breaths, inhaling gratitude, you will exhale bliss.
Aloha.

Time and Hawaiian Time

Here at the beginning, it is useful to acknowledge the Hawaiian way of knowing time, which is so far across the sea from clock time. Hawaiian time, in the Halau, is vertical. Wherever you are, be it O'ahu, Minneapolis, or Toronto, living in the Aloha Spirit is living in vertical time. Having a Lomilomi treatment seems on the surface like a spa vacation for an hour. Yet people long to savor and continue the freedom and pleasure of their vacations or massage even in the midst of the workaday world. Living in an awareness of the reality of vertical time can fulfill that longing.

What is vertical time? Vertical time means no deadlines, no fixed schedules. Vertical time means freedom, kindness, unity, humility, patience, alertness. Vertical time we all share with God. Healing may be outside our comfort zone or boundaries. If so, a part of those boundaries are linear time. If healing were inside our comfort zone, we would already be healed. Thinking that a trip to the islands is a vacation to a destination is linear time. Believing that a trip to the islands is an inner journey to wholeness is vertical time.

HARRY: The ancient ones believed that all time is now, that we are each creators of our lifestyle and its conditions. We created who we are and everything that becomes a part of our lives. Any situation we might find ourselves in is brought about by us in learning the many pathways of life. Our situations are not the results of a judgment of our actions. But who we become is caused by our thoughts and choices.

To Hawaiians, linear time is the dream of commonality that all minds share. The Halau Uhane Lomilomi Lapaʻau is the journey of conscious partnership between you and your emotional body. It is the expression of the Hawaiians' premise and perception of the world around them—that we are in linear and vertical time.

We all live in the linear time. It is the watch on your arm determining your schedule. Vertical time, on the other hand, is that connection with the Higher Self. The Hawaiian knows, and we want you to know, how to emotionally invest in Spirit: the *Auʻmakua*, the infinite mind of you, the light of the presence of God in you. (This will be explored further in chapter two.)

GARNETTE: The Greeks called timelessness "no-time" or *Kairos*. Clock time is *Kronos*, chronological time. Working nine to five is linear time, then. Vertical time is free of the clock, a vacation from boundaries to the bliss of timelessness—God's time, not past, present, or future, but Paʻa, the now.

HARRY: We call that now time Pa'a. Lomilomi, like surfing, is both a vertical and linear time experience. Both activities require the skill of navigating personal emotions, while moving in unity with energy. The only navigation available to guide you is truth in the Spirit. The task of maneuvering a Lomilomi treatment and maneuvering through the center of a wave requires the Lomilomi giver and the surfer to receive information and grace from the Higher Self. This is why these are both vertical and linear experiences.

A Lomilomi session is about the moments when a person's vibration is raised vertically to that Pa'a, the now, that presence of God in us, for maybe two to three seconds. Then all the rest of the session before and after is entertainment, anchoring the feeling of Pa'a, the now, into the person's experience.

Harry's Story: The Vertical Time Experience

When I was eleven years old, I stood on a surfboard and went into the waves. And I felt oneness with God, time, the waves, the ocean, the sky, with all. Surfing became my religion for a while. I exulted in vertical time. It was no-time, yet vibrantly alive, and I was one with surfing. Hawaiians really value the emotional presence of our bodies in vertical time. Again I say, vertical time is what we all share with God in the present. When we crack the pattern that causes illness, there is happiness in a nanosecond, in the Pa'a, the now.

So when you swim into the meanings of Hawaiian words, relax, have fun. Remember the less definitions, the more space. Emotional maturity is the fortitude to know yourself better. Look into the home of your mind to see where you live. Your mind can direct the force of power of gratitude to your body. Say:

My body knows how to take care of this body. My body sends signals, pain and pleasure signals.

Preparing the Path

As we begin to explore this realm of Hawaiian body work healing, we do first things first. We prepare the path. We already have

Aloha, the presence of God within us, and we know we can move at will between linear time into the Pa'a, the now, of vertical time. Where do we find the path?

Opportunities are given to you in the space of the Halau. The tradition of the Halau is that touch medicine is learned in both vertical and linear time. Experience is based on the format. Therefore, be quiet and listen first in order to find the path to healing. The way to see or feel and then know what is inside the space of Lomilomi is through the traditional style.

Harry's Story: The Uhane Lineage, the People of Uhane

I am in the lineage of the namesake Uhane. The second of four in Pa'a, the now, here, with this generation. The Uhane can be traced in the *Kumulipu*, an ancient chant of four thousand generations of history that is in the kahuna's keeping and that takes about three days and three nights of continuous speaking. The *Kumulipu*, in Hawaiian, means "genesis."

From the beginning of our group-mind intention to Pa'a, the now, the Kumulipu records every clan of the original few people and the ancestral progression of each namesake as it has grown, then matured, then been completely destroyed in the genocide. Hawaiians have been experiencing genocide since Captain Cook's arrival in 1778.

The Kumulipu, according to the learnings I carry, is a chant that bends through time into a circle of completion. The genocide of the Hawaiian nationality is bemoaned as terrorism on the face of each native Hawaiian. The terrorism is the destruction of our lands and culture. On the inside, found in the light of the Hawaiian DNA, is the knowing that however much we are grieving this genocide, it proves our time here with the mother, *Mauna Loa*, is completed. We have achieved the circle of perfection, which is what we Hawaiians came to this Earth to do.

The word *kahuna* is a verb, not a noun. The Hawaiian knows this because the Hawaiian feels the Kumulipu inside. The DNA presence of the Hawaiian was, is, and will be the holder of the truth,

Directions to Preparing the Path's Landscape

In Lomilomi, the physical is a tiny bit.

Lomilomi is a mindset, a perspective that generates healing.

Say, I am plenty. I love me. I am enough.

Lomilomi gives the body potency, vitality, and rejuvenation.

Lomilomi is not what you expect, it's what you feel.

Lomilomi is four techniques that simply can be unveiled.

Lomilomi is a gift of Spirit to humanity.

Lomilomi is emotional evolution.

There will be no tests. Nobody fails.

Therein is your growth.

until the truth seed is ready to expand. The culture has done too much and has had too much done to it on this Earth. Our mother the Earth is *Moana*. The Hawaiian culture is dying, as will Mother Earth. Moana not only dies, but also comes to completion, to resolution, giving us freedom to move through to higher or parallel fields of consciousness. The Hawaiian culture, like all circle-based cultures, is lovingly leaving us jewels of ever-expanding knowledge.

I was born in 1958. In that time, there were three Uhane: me, my father, and my grandfather—Harry Uhane Ekau Jim our namesake source. Grandfather was Uhane clan from Maui. He was *Hanai*, meaning that he was adopted by the Ekau Ohana (the Ekau family).

His birth mother, my great-grandmother, was Hina ha Uhane of Hana, Maui. Her name, *Hina ha Uhane*, is a tribute in the feminine context and means "the healing sister of Pele." Pele is known worldwide as the fire goddess of Kilauea. In the canonization of the seven sisters of Pele, the Kumulipu accounts Hina, the gray one, the energy of the mist of the forest mountains. The underside of the *Lehua* leaf in the mountains is *hina*, a mix between silver and green. We know that the realm of the patriarch in the place of healing is the hina, the Ha, the breath of the spirit of the healing sister of Pele, that immortal being Hina Uhane.

But it is critical to understand that the name's tribute is not to the personality or deity of Hina, nor to the noun. The tribute is to the energy of the verb *hina*.

Harry Uhane Ekau Jim was my father's father. When my paternal grandfather was born, he was the end of the line. He was the only Uhane left. Then upon his twenty-seventh year he came to the island of Kauai, and my father was born through his mother, Marilyn Manoi. I was very close to grandfather Uhane.

From these grandparents came my father, Harold Uhane Jim. His Uhane connects the lineage of the Manoi clan, who trace their Kumulipu to keepers of the mountain known as Kahili. This Kahili mountain is on Kauai, near the south Koloa area, separate from Lihue crater and other mountain ranges. It is the place where the people Mu were received by Moana, where Mother Earth greeted these Pleiadians. Again, the tribute in the name *Kahili* is not to mountain the noun, but the verb, the energy, of the mountain.

I myself landed (was born) on Moana on the island of Kauai. If you ever landed on Kauai, you know you have come to a full and regal expression of Moana. Kauai is the oldest in the chain of islands and the purest expression of the mind at peace. She is an artist's palette of greens and blues that splash open your being, all in a sensual envelope of perpetually vitalized air.

I came through this time near my father's twenty-seventh year on Kauai. My mother, Janet Marie Desilva Jim, was born on Kauai and not with lineage to the Kumulipu. She was the daughter of a couple from Madeira, also an island, off the coast of Portugal. Her twentieth year gave her the third Uhane-to-be—me.

In my twentieth year, the last Uhane of his generation, Grandpa, passed. In my twenty-seventh year came the new third Uhane of Pa'a, the now—our son Kapono Uhane Isaiah—on Kauai through his mother Sila Lehua, granddaughter of Papa David Kaonohiokala Bray. Their linage carries the kahuna seed on through to the kahuna, the Seeing Eye of the Sun. This kahunas' clan is the shaper and manager of the belief systems. Keola-Uhane David Jim, or the fourth Uhane, came to Sila Lehua and myself in my thirty-fourth year—this one lands on the island of Hawaii. Now there are four Uhane.

There has been for four thousand generations Uhane in the seed (or the egg). This the Kumulipu recounts.

Our link—Sila and I—is five children: Keola, Keani, Kapono, Kala'e, and Leinani. Not all of the children are kahuna the noun, but all have kahuna the verb. *Keola* means the one who holds health; *Keani Kalaheiwa*, the sweet breeze of the mountain fern; *Kapono*, the rightful and balanced; *Kala'e*, calm and clear; and *Leinani*, heaven's garland.

I took the challenge to be a Lomilomi giver when I was three, although I was young. By the time I was age four, family and friends were asking me to do healing touch. When you take the challenge to be a Lomilomi giver, you will radiate healing. People who receive will feel better. Your power as a witness of grace receiving gratitude comes from the shift in your belief system. (This will be explored further in chapter four.)

Kahunas do not tell how to shift the belief system into deep understanding, but instead do Lomilomi. This is because kahunas don't want to hold you back from embracing all of vertical time. When you find it yourself, you will own it. Don't tell, show; don't say, do. If kahunas tell, they divert you from your own discovery and your own ability to swim deep, alone with Spirit only.

I'o: The Hawk

To Hawaiians *God* is a verb, an action—not a noun or a name. Emotions, too, are actions. God's motive for creation is so that we can experience life more fully and get to know ourselves better. God was motivated to create so that we might find/achieve the ultimate expression of emotional maturity.

In the Eastern religions there is no word for God, a concept so huge. In the *I Ching*, to Hinduism ultimately, and to Buddhism, God is a force. To Hawaiians also, God is pure nondualism in the ultimate. For teaching purposes, the highest representation of the ancient ones—so omniscient, omnipresent, and omnipotent—was the hawk, I'o, soaring over the highest volcanoes. Understand this, it is critical to healing. Lomilomi empowers the God in you. Our job as Lomilomi givers is to be the witness of the receiver's work, to resolve and absolve. Everyone can experience the state of Pa'a, the now, vertical no-time. You have already experienced it, but with Lomilomi you learn to enter it at will. Enter and exit into your Higher Self as you Lomilomi your life. You have the techniques in you; bring them out. You have the capacity to trust yourself. This is what it takes to be a healer. I know every one of you, and I love you.

Kathleen's Healing Story

I had suffered a particularly nefarious breakup with a fiancé, and I was tired of thinking, feeling, and talking. My dear friend Helen suggested I go for a massage by this Lomilomi master she had just met and with whom she had an incredible experience. Perfect, I thought—have him rub it out. I had no idea what Lomilomi was. But I didn't care. I trusted Helen implicitly.

Well, it was six sessions later before I got that massage.

Harry, immediately perceiving the crumpled condition I was in, preceded to break with (what I believe as a Western) convention; he disclosed that he had met my ex and his (new) girlfriend, and he gave me perspective on the situation. It was like conversing with an auntie but way better. He talked, breathed, and changed me back to health within about six weeks. It would have taken me a couple of years on my own, I believe. Then he began to take me places psychologically and spiritually I had never been before.

I became intrigued with Lomilomi and took Harry's class. After the first class, I immediately scheduled a private session—still never having had a massage—and asked him to demonstrate all the techniques he would be showing us in class so I would know what they were supposed to feel like. "Oh, I'm not done with you yet" was his response, and he gave me a massage that had me walking six inches off the ground for a week.

I particularly enjoyed the conversations we had about spirituality in the classes. No dogma, no protocol. So simple and basic are the concepts of the self and "other," they were hard to grasp—we live our lives with such expected, perceived, and real complication. I do not have the vocabulary to express succinctly what I learned, and it is difficult to transmit verbally. It seems that so much of what Harry taught us is a way of feeling, being, perceiving, transmitting our spirituality—or allowing our spirituality to be transmitted. There is a higher order, and Harry is directly connected to it. And the feeling of his connection made me want to be connected too. Harry makes the connection easy.

I especially enjoy how much we laugh—in class and in private sessions. This is the state our mind, hearts, and spirits need to be in—to succor the often wrenching complexity of our daily existence. And again, "succor" implies a patch, and is the wrong word. Existing in the proper mental-spiritual state allows us to bend and sway with the turmoil, to roll with the punches and not be broken by them—but more importantly, to revel in the multitudinous gifts that abound if we are receptive to perceive them.

WHAT YOU CAN EXPECT AS A LOMILOMI GIVER

- *Your belief system will change.*

- *Your power as a witness of grace receiving gratitude will come through the shift of your belief system.*

- *You will acquire the skill of shape-shifting energy in the body and moving it out of the body.*

- *Your comfort zone will expand.*

- *You will be able to shape the space connecting the body to the healing window.*

- *Your emotional body will evolve so as to communicate with you.*

- *You will radiate healing.*

- *You will grasp your capacity to reverse the polarity paradigm of your self-trust.*

- *You will manage energy through the three states of consciousness: asleep, awake, and aware.*

CHAPTER TWO

The Triune Self
and the Meaning in Aloha

In this chapter we explore esoteric meanings of Hawaiian words and realms. But first, here's how to learn to swim in the deep ocean—Hawaiian style.

Harry's Story

When I was three years old, I wanted to learn to swim in the deep water. We were living on Kauai island. My dad took me over to the ocean one Sunday morning, early. We looked at the vastness of the ocean, and I was suddenly afraid. I was three and small, the ocean was ancient and endless.

Instead of taking me in the water, my dad hunkered down to show me the pebbles in the sand. He showed me how to let the sand run through my fingers, sorting out the pretties. We found some *pu'ka* shells. Those little creatures from the reef are so valuable to collect and sell as necklaces. They are round like coins, white and purple; we pierce a hole in them and string hundreds for one necklace. One daughter is doing this now, living on the beach, gathering the pu'ka shells to make necklaces.

So my dad and I rambled over the sand, poking around, looking at rocks. He told me about the shellfish. And that the ocean is my friend. I wanted to rush right into the water then. But he said, next time.

When we came back, he walked into the warm water up to his toes, and I followed eagerly. Then to the ankles, then the knees, until finally, when it was deep to me, he sank down and swam under me so I was on his back. We went out into the deeper waters of our friend the ocean. Then he floated apart, and I kept on swimming.

I too give my children the support they need so they can swim into their lives. That's why we live in Buffalo now. So my children can have the experience and attend schools here. When they can swim on their own, my wife and I will return to live full time in Hawaii. We still have our houses there, our families. This is a story of learning how to quietly live with Spirit. My father, my two sons, and myself are the only Hawaiians named Uhane, Spirit of Will.

Life is good.

How Does Aloha Move from a Greeting to the Light?

Every Hawaiian word has seven fields of meaning. Come, let us swim through these levels as we meet together.

Aloha is a word where each syllable is a sacred sound. Each sound thus has its own esoteric meaning. In the case of *Ah*, it is an abbreviation of God's name. God's full name is not spoken by Hawaiians just as in Judaism or Advaita. With reverence for the ultimate unknowable, we do not say God's name, only an abbreviation. We say "ahhh," the sound of appreciation of the breath. Old-time mainland physicians used to place a wooden stick in the patient's mouth and direct, "Say ahhh." Perhaps they had been to Hawaii and learned the healing sound of an extended A. Relax in the peace of God in the sound of ahhh. It means the radiation of divine energy in the multidimensional universe. Say "ahhh." Rest. Now you have called upon God for healing.

Aloha will become a beloved and familiar term to you as you swim through this book of the Aloha Spirit. *Alo* means "the presence of God with us" or "love certainly" and *ha* means breath. So one meaning of Aloha is "the breath of God is in our presence."

Sometimes people think it is ironic that the English language only has one word for love, and that is *love*, while the Inuits have more than seventy-three for snow. In Russian there are multiple words for degrees of love. So, too, in Hawaiian there are many definitions for the one word, *Aloha*, all meaning "love." Some of the dictionary words for *Aloha* are "caring," "affection," "compassion," "mercy," "sympathy," "pity," "kindness," "regard with affection," even "to desire." Also, of course, "hello," "good-bye," "farewell." Then there is Garnette's favorite: *aloha-ai* denoting "consumed by divine love," an all-consuming love, a state of bliss such as the one we savor in the poetry of Rumi.

Yet *Aloha* with *pe* can mean "alas." Curiously, until you think about it, *Aloha* can also mean "to die": *Ka alo* or *Ma alo* means "to pass over," "to cross over," to die. (In Harry's next book, he will tell you more about the Hawaiian belief in the continuum of life and the energy of Aloha.)

Yes, the word *Aloha* means many things: hello, good-bye, welcome love (in various degrees and forms), alas, and to pass/cross over, to die/transition.

Now let's go through each letter of *Aloha* to intuit the word's seventh and most secret meaning.

Unveiling the Structure of Aloha

As there are seven rays of light in rainbows, there are also seven planes or realms. Each plane holds a distinct purpose and vibration. The first level is called the Gate of Heaven, or the opening door to all the other fields. Aloha as a greeting is like that gate, opening the vibration in order to manifest energy.

Elements of light distinctly characterize the energies of the fields. None are specific to healing, but without that knowing, you would have a blind landscape to manifesting the spiritual. The theory that all the gods are dead and represent only a concept of the duality is false. To the Hawaiians the gods represent intelligences of vibrations of energy. *Lono*, the god of rain, as an entity is really a cache of intelligence. That intelligence is in the realm of sound. Since God's sound has made us manifest in the physical world, the intent of God is granted power through the human voicing of Aloha. That which holds the vibration of that intelligence is Lono.

Healing permeates Hawaii because people say *Aloha*. Words hold power.

Hold that concept of "the Breath of God is in our Presence" through saying *Aloha*. The highest experience of the concept and power of Aloha seems to disengage mainlanders from their groundedness in the mundane and the linear and sprinkle Lono's love like rain. Exposing the power of Lono to the spirit of the newcomers gives them access to rejuvenation. What is such renewal? The simple, childlike ability of being in the right now.

The old tourist greeting is "Aloha, Aloha." The first Aloha is cheery. The second is underlining its emphasis. A third time is silence, which really means the traveler can really feel the gasp of wonderment and release. Because they have attachments, the sound of *Aloha* can hit right at the heart, which brings Lono to aliveness now. Then they look around, they notice everyone else and become aligned with them; they giggle with emotion, and they say for some unpredictable reason they see people are happy. That's the sound of *Aloha* among them as a blessing.

The old missionaries believed God had personality, an ego. Missionaries believed their god generated power from victims, martyrdoms, war games. Then the Jungians said that these personalities are archetypes of God. That's not the secret of *Huna*, which is that the gods represent intelligences of vibrations of energy. The school of Harry's lineage of kahunas dissects how these intelligences of sound/vibrations are to the icon of Lono and how that intelligence of sound can manifest miracles of healing. That's a piece cloaked in the word *Aloha*.

Sila's grandfather, kahuna Papa Bray lived outside the victim/ martyr concept. Papa Bray said, "Aloha to the Hawaiians of old is God in us. It means, 'Come forward, be in unity and harmony with your real self, God, and mankind. Be honest, be truthful, patient, kind to all forms of life, and humble.' "

A   *Ala* is watchful alertness. Consciousness of all seeing awareness. Omniscience.

L   *Lokahi* is working with unity. In the eyes of God, no one is above another, all are connected. In unity, one sees God in all form.

O   *Oiaio* is truthful honesty, authenticity. (Papa Bray says O means that humanity can also experience unreality, misinterpretation that leads to negative emotions and wrong actions, which turn into unhappiness, illness, and death.) O knows that what you are feeling inside is manifested outside.

H   *Haahaa* is humility. *Ha* is breath or Spirit; *haahaa* is the emotion of Spirit having a human experience.

A   *Ahonui* patient perseverance. The knowing that gravity and attention are the same thing.

"This is the secret teaching of Aloha," says Papa Bray. "These five letters of Aloha are a set of principles that support the kahuna in their work, whether it is building canoes or healing a body or navigating the open ocean. It is all the same condition of focus and effort."

Now you glimpse the subtlety of the true Hawaiian language. It's amorphous. It is not directly translatable into English, although the missionaries tried by changing or bending sounds to fit English. Each syllable has layers and layers of meaning. Each layer depends on the subtle sound of the consciousness of the speaker and the nuances of an oral tradition. When the missionaries came, they heard the fluidity of the Hawaiian language, but they came to it with their boxed-in thinking.

Aloha, the breath of God is in our presence, includes seeing the nuances of the breathing, not only the words. To Hawaiians it was an insult to hide the chest so breathing could not be viewed. The main conversation was nonverbal breathing together in harmony, as much as the sounds exchanged. When Captain Cook and the missionaries came swabbed in thick wool suits and layers of long underwear and confining shirts and shoes, the Hawaiians thought they were trying to conceal their breathing patterns and so must have trickery on their minds. The newcomers tried to enclose this openness of language and breath into their own culture, their formula. Thus the hard anchor sounds of the consonants *b*, *t*, *m*, and *k* were imposed onto the subtle and easygoing vowels. It was like covering beautiful bodies with heavy cloth. So when you swim into the meanings of the Hawaiian words, relax, have fun. Remember the fewer definitions, the more space. The less clothing, the more relaxation. So laugh now. Just sit and laugh for a while. We have plenty of space for Aloha! Breathe in harmony like the breezes of the trade winds.

Triune Human Being

As a Lomilomi giver, you are the least important person in the room. Lomilomi is all about Uhane, the Spirit of Will, which embraces the receiver. You are not your body, your mind, your history, or even your future. As the giver you are saying to the receiver, "I am not afraid of your pain. I know it; I hear its voice. Together we will release this cry of pain into your emotionally mature voice, the Uhane."

However, this does not mean that the receiver's pain does not exist. You are real—more real than your present reality, more solid and more spirit than outer circumstances reflect.

Here's how Hawaiian kahunas understand the complex physical psyche of a human being. They use three terms—*Auʻmakua*,

Uhane, and *Unihipili*—for the triune human being. Greet these important words and bring their essence into your awareness. Breathe them in. They are the triune self, who you really are. Once you have mastered these Hawaiian terms you can better understand the methodology of Lomilomi. For Lomilomi shifts the energies locked in the body by unlocking the triune aspects into flow.

The body's prime directive is to love and serve you and tell you what is going on with it. The body is a communication tool for travel and entertainment of Spirit on this plane. Physical pain is the body telling you that you have disharmony. The body knows more about healing than your mind does. Healing is creating a new thought pattern in your body. As a Lomilomi giver, enjoy being the witness to the healing. It's fun to be the witness as you expand and partake in the vibration building. In Lomilomi, the giver directs the traffic in the receiver's mind, body, and spirit. Touch is spirit-to-spirit communication. But in some sessions you will never touch at all; it may be all breath work. The giver is comforting and securing to the receiver's body. The giver is making some room in the receiver's body so things (pain, blocks) that need to move on out can. The giver is witnessing and knowing "I AM still here with you" as the receiver heals from inside out.

OPPORTUNITY

Breath is essential in Lomilomi for uniting the three selves to the whole. Breathe in a complete cycle—in through the nose, out through the mouth—thirty times. This is a simple practice of intent that unleashes mana loa (power, energy).

Unleashing Mana

Mana is an important word in Polynesia, although it is also recognizable worldwide. *Mana* is pronounced with a long *ah*, exactly like it is in manna, the word for the bread the Hebrews gathered by grace in the Sinai desert. Mana is subtle energy, yet it carries a power. Think of the Force in the *Star Wars* films, then shift it from wars to healing. Mana is integral to understanding the Hawaiian and to practicing Temple Lomilomi.

This energy, which is power, is known in many cultures—in China as *chi*, India as *prana*, and Japan as *ki*. To Hawaiians mana accumulates in the solar plexus. Hawaiians treasure bulk and girth as signs of stored mana. Mana is relaxed, not forced, energy. Mana flows and creates ease. Think of the laughing Buddha statue, HoTi, whose big belly it is good fortune to rub. The Hindu swamis, such as Swami Nityanandaji Maharaj and Paramahamsa Yogananda, eat practically nothing, yet carry large bellies of stored energy, or *shakti*.

Dividing the Water of the Three-Self Vessel of the Physical Body

First understand, the Asian chakra system has one, two, three, four, five, six, and so on chakras in order. To the Polynesians the energy centers are more like the infinity symbol with the intersection meeting at the solar plexus—the heart, which is the core of the energy system. So the High Self is from above the crown to the bottom of the heart. The Middle Self is from the brow to the bottom of the heart. The Low Self is the bottom of the heart. The form is that of the infinity symbol, yet amorphous. It is approximate, indescribable in physical terms because it's Spirit, not a physical location.

To talk to your triune self in the body, which is your temple, you may *pu'le* (pray) to divide the waters from the Unihipili directed by the Uhane to the Au'makua. Each morning from your will, direct your unconscious to pray to your High Self. In the evening during meditation, pray your gratitude to your triune self. How? First understand the wisdom, love, and strength of the amorphous triune self.

Au'makua

The High Self, the superconscious, "All are One," the great "I Am" within, the Wise Parent

• *Aspects of the Au'makua, the Pure Light Within*

To Hawaiians, the Divine Source is pure nondualism that cannot have attributes or be described. It is still essential to remember all Hawaiian words have several layers. Here we are talking about the finest essence of Au'makua. Within the triune human self radiates the Au'makua, the Pure Light within, the Presence of God within, which does have nameable and knowable aspects. The wise Au'makua is rooted in the heart and located in the chakra center that is above the crown. The Au'makua guards, nurtures, and shines light on seeds of potential within each individual. The Au'makua, the God flame in an individual, but not God, is the guardian and completely trustworthy parental spirit, as well as the connection to the Source and to the higher, ethereal realms. Parental yet androgynous, composed of equally balanced male and female energy, this wise Au'makua produces attainments and miracles. The Au'makua converts God energy into Mana, power on the physical plane. The Au'makua is an expression of a person's own perfection.

The wise Au'makua has the power to recognize causes, fixations, possessions, or identifications while being judgment free, as it is not capable of mistakes, which require judging. The Au'makua requires invitation, and thus it can be pu'le, prayed to; yet it cannot and will not interfere in the conscious mind's free will. The wise Au'makua will do no harm even if asked to do so. The Au'makua possesses the power to predict and affect the future to change a person's path/life. The Au'makua does not allow negative thinking (if we choose negativity, the Au'makua does not accept it).

The Au'makua is omniscient, sees all past and future in vertical time.

The Au'makua in the triune self-person is all forgiving.

Uhane

The Middle Self, the will of spirit, conscious will; adult

• Aspects of the Uhane, the Conscious Spirit of Will

The Uhane is located in the third eye at the brow and extends to the heart area. The loving Uhane converts mana into thinking and feeling. The Uhane takes thought-forms from Unihipili and transmits to the Au'makua, the Light world.

The loving Uhane is the emotionally strong, mature consciousness and voice that plants seeds of Light in the Unihipili, the wondrous unconscious, at will. This mature conscious mind, the Uhane, has free will to deny the Presence, or even the existence, of Au'makua, the High Self. The Uhane does not suspend the illusion of separation because of free will. Yet Uhane sustains the entertainment of free will, which is your "personal" life. The Uhane is not related to the Freudian concept of the ego; while comparisons don't really work, the Uhane, the Spirit of Will, is closer to the Asian concept of higher will, *buddhi*, an egoless state. The Uhane directs action requests to the Unihipili to communicate with the Au'makua for the greater good of the triune self.

Unihipili

The Low Self, the unconscious, the collective unconscious; childlike.

• Aspects of Unihipili, the Wondrous Unconscious Mind

The Unihipili is located in the solar plexus. It controls the supply and use of mana loa. It is innocent, and it loves and protects the High Self. The Unihilipi is linear and literal, bound by time.

The Uhane wills the Unihipili to send seeds of light to the Au'makua. The Unihilipi stores memories in the brain and the bone that the kahunas know how to wash out. The unconscious Unihipili is the domain of emotions, which can suddenly pop out or bushwhack the person from the unconscious, as well as furnish bliss. The Unihipili organizes memories in horizontal-linear time and in vertical time. The Unihipili represses memories that are negative by crystallizing them in the body. One of the Unihipili's jobs is to protect the adult Uhane from bad and hurt feelings while holding the blueprint of the body's capacity to function perfectly.

Another task of the Unihipili as the unconscious is to preserve the body so as to maintain the body's integrity no matter what happens to it. The Unihipili is extremely moral and follows directions from Au'makua. The Unihipili loves the Uhane unconditionally and is loyal to the Uhane unconditionally.

The Unihipili controls and monitors physical and telepathic perceptions. The Unihipili generates, stores, distributes, and transmits mana energy at the direction of the Au'makua. The Unihipili, like the child it is and always will be, responds with instinct and habit to situations. It requires repetition as its food, so repeated pu'le is good.

The Unihilipi supports curiosity, naturally seeing more, discovering more, in a childlike way. Like the innocent, it responds to symbols and speaks in symbols as well, for the Unihipili takes everything personally. And it operates on a path of least resistance.

The Unihipili gives away its free will to the Uhane, the adult of the triune being. The Unihipili regularly sends thought-forms from the dense physical world to Au'makua's light world, which appreciates the partnership with the Unihipili. The Au'makua parent loves the creative playfulness of the child Unihipili. The parent gives all it can, nurturing the child unconditionally.

So now you can understand the triune inner realms in each person. All three aspects are within each person and connected to each and every other person in partnership with the greater good. Au'makua, Uhane, Unihipili. Parent, adult, child. Superconscious, conscious, unconscious.

As a Lomilomi giver, you will be in contact with your own three realms and the three realms of receivers. Remember the Au'makua in you is one with the Au'makua of all others at the same time and thus is omniscient. Only the Supreme Absolute, however, is omnipotent. To the ancient Hawaiians, the higher beings beyond the three realms in the physical body were unknowable, all-powerful, and in comparison to the tiny human being, formless in totality. The Supreme was beyond the moon, beyond the stars, beyond the sun, beyond all known and understanding. The humility of not knowing, yet knowing, is the gift of the Hawaiian's understanding the pure, nondualistic eternal.

An Anonymous Healing Story

In 2001, before my pulmonary-artery cancer diagnosis, I was in a near-fatal car crash and had to be removed with the Jaws of Life. The accident wasn't my fault. One person died. I went into a deep and debilitating post-traumatic stress (PTS) syndrome. I tried everything Western medicine could offer, including antidepressants and counseling, but nothing relieved the anxiety I lived under.

Then in three different ways, I heard about Harry. First, I was at a lecture, and somebody I didn't know walked by, pointed, and said, "There's a real Hawaiian kahuna. Go see him." Then my therapist recommended I check Harry out. Last, I went to an open house; Harry was there, too. To me, it was Spirit showing me to pay attention.

OPPORTUNITY

Four deep in-and-out breath cycles, directed to the solar plexus, consciously sends energy to Au'makua from Unihipili, which creates in Uhane and reflects in your world.

So I made an appointment. It has been an incredible journey. Harry has a great deal of experience in treating PTS with Vietnam veterans. He knew immediately that my adrenal glands were stuck open. He made me believe I was going to be OK. My condition did get worse before it got better, but getting better was a wonderful thing.

Then I developed a persistent cough that wouldn't go away, and I had a shortness of breath. So I had a chest x-ray. They found an inoperable tumor in my lungs that was the size of my heart. Harry introduced me to Alice Mammoser, a gifted iridologist, and both of them saw me coming out the other end. The people I needed, and enormous amounts of energy, were sent into my life. When I doubted it, Harry reminded me. Now I believe you cannot get through cancer unless you strongly know you are going to get through it. Alice gave me, and I exaggerate only slightly, about fifty thousand vitamins, herbs, and homeopathics. Harry worked on the energy part of it and said he was doing flushing on the cellular level. By February, five months later, the tumor had shrunk in half, and I had lung surgery. As of April I am cancer free, and I know I will remain cancer free, because Harry said so. Harry does not say stuff that's not true. He called every step.

For people who understand, cancer can be a gift and life can change. I don't even know who I am going to be, now that I have survived cancer, but I know it will be spectacular, incredible.

The operation did some nerve damage to my left hand, messed up what I did for a living. Now Harry has been working on my hand, and it's range of motion has fully come back.

I think Harry came to Buffalo for me. But it wasn't just him who helped me. There were many, many invisible beings in his treatment room. [She is talking about the Halau guardians.] His work is a vessel that serves a much higher source. Sometimes when I lay on the table I would feel them over my face when Harry was working down at my feet. The fact that Harry came into my life is miraculous. Now I sit quietly and give gratitude for the grace received—grace that comes from so many planes, energy so overwhelming. I've always been energy sensitive and now the awareness of grace bowls me over with gratitude.

And I cannot have pessimism; it knocks me off course. If I go into faltering, Harry would remind me. Lomilomi gave me strength on the mental, physical, and energetic level to learn to breathe with one lung, to practice walking from one end of the house to another, to watch my hair grow back. Now I am in as much control as humanly possible. Sometime I just throw things up to the Universe, and the Universe will take and carry the anxiety away. I learned from Harry just to float in the Universe, to trust that Higher Self, the Au'makua, the part of the self that is one with the Universe. I can do that now. I am eager to see what's next.

CHAPTER THREE

Creating Space for Healing

Aloha Aloha nui nui.

Nui Nui means extremely good. Adding *nui* to Aloha, "the Breath of God is in our presence," takes us into the deep valley of healing where all is good.

Harry and I met at the botanical gardens in Lackawanna, New York, one summer morning. The dew was just drying off the grass. He settled down on that grass just as if on soft beach sand. Gardeners were buzzing around, as were the bees. One young man zoomed by on a golf cart with a large tree in the back, waving towards our sun-dappled spot. "Oh, a three-year-old banana tree," Harry said, pointing. "So Hawaiian." Our space for work was created in that simple act. Suddenly, it seemed as if old Hawaii was our location. It was a quiet Sunday morning in the northeast United States, yet the garden aromas, the gentle wind, and the easygoing approach we were taking created a private world. It was the perfect setting for discussing the Hawaiian creation story and the concept of the technique Creating Space.

The Kahunas' Healing Heritage

GARNETTE: Tell us more about the kahunas, please. Are all kahunas healers?

HARRY: First, you would need to know there are several different paths of kahunas. My lineage, and my energy, is of the healing kahunas of Lomilomi, touch medicine. This medicine comes by direct grace. It is the medicine of comfort, sanctity, and safety. It is also the medicine of witness.

GARNETTE: You are using the word *medicine* in the sense of "good medicine," as the First Americans, the native people here, do.

HARRY: Yes, as in "good medicine" or "bad medicine." Not technological medicine. That's an important distinction. For these principles of medicine are of the energy all kahunas invite into their power. The mana comes from vertical time, not linear. Healing power comes from the field of the rainbow vibrations of the Halau Guardians which is God's Light.

GARNETTE: When you say *field*, you are referring to the higher realms or the range of responsibility?

HARRY: The collective energy field of the Guardians of Light and the shamans, the kahunas, and gifted spiritual healers were separate from day-to-day tribal binds, or *kapu*. These binds or boundaries were the social glue and lubricants to help the people in their journey through linear time. Healers do not have to have that physical structure or psychological/emotional structure the people do. They have a spiritual structure, a purpose apart from tribal boundaries. The healing kahunas had to connect with the guardians.

GARNETTE: So kahunas were recognized as keepers of the spiritual powers for the people. What was their relationship with the rulers, the royalty?

HARRY: The *Ali'i* were the monarchs. The kahunas served them and the people as the advisors and healers. If the tribes did not cherish their healers, they would lose their power to emotionally evolve.

Hawaiians were not only physically separate on their islands in the remote Pacific Ocean, but they also were a different and separate people from the rest of the human race. Hawaiians' creation stories differ in that their ancestors were the ones that did not leave paradise; they brought it—their home—with them to the islands from interstellar space. This makes a huge difference in the basic belief system. Hawaiians had not alienated themselves from their Source Guardians.

GARNETTE: They did not leave the Garden of Eden then?

HARRY: That is a code for leaving Paradise. Our stories tell us by oral tradition that Hawaiians came from the star cluster *Honu*, which you call the Dog Star, in the Pleiades. They came to live in the land we call *Mu* which evolved into the nation we know of as Hawaii. They lived gracefully there with the Aloha that permeated all life. For eons, kahunas have traveled the seas, navigated by the stars, irrigated the fields with water, and lived by the oral tradition. Eventually, for some people the connection was lost; others, kahunas, however, remember because of the secret teachings passed from healer to healer. This is why the keepers of the secrets have the ability to directly contact the community of light, the Kumulipu genealogy of the Source Guardians. They are one with the community of light beings, the brothers and sisters of Light. These beings envelop the vitality of the Light. The Kahuna way of seeing becomes the fullness of vertical time within. The Kumulipu genealogy chant traces our origins. It takes a full three days and three nights to chant it using the deep and low chant voice. It begins with a sound like *I'o—I-e-o*—and then the sound reversed. As you move through these sounds, the vibration's rising in both the people and the environment. I begin my workshops with these chants. As you chant, you are saying at the first level, "I am that of the I'o hawk, holding omniscience and omnipotence by the currency of grace receiving gratitude."

GARNETTE: Will you be saying more about grace?

HARRY: Throughout the whole book. Grace is thundering. That's why it was important to put the ancient glyph on the cover of the book. It means Thundering Grace.

Recording the Star Connection

GARNETTE: Masaru Emoto, author of *The Hidden Messages in Water* and *The True Power of Water*, says that water did not originate on this planet but came to it in the form of ice comets.

So too people came—people came with extrasensory perceptions, people whose descendents are intermingled with us today. People like the Hawaiians, who remember their connections to the stars and are adepts with cosmic gifts. Hawaiians did not leave Paradise; they created it here just like it was at home. So this knowing of Paradise differs with that of the missionaries, who arrived primed with teachings of exile, longing, guilt, and fear. The missionaries' ideas actually were opposite of the Hawaiian knowledge that home is where they are. Therein lies the kahuna's power for healing. Basically missionaries saw God as a force outside of us and Hawaiians still see God as a force that resides within.

To begin understanding from whence the healing kahunas' power comes, know that there are at least two sources.

HARRY: The material form is only one source. Also there is the pure source. If people had no attachments or judgments or belief systems, we would see only sparks of light above their chairs. But people do have belief systems. These belief systems create their bodies and minds, but their core is still Light.

It is the work of Lomilomi to envelop the guardians within the patient. This sounds esoteric, and it is, but it is also common sense. Auntie Mary used to say healing is 80 percent spirit, 20 percent touch. Once she had a patient come to her with a painful hiatal hernia. She told me that her work was to comfort the disagreement at the top of the sternum. She said touch would help, but really the source was the patient's lack of love she had with her husband. So the work of Lomilomi is to go back to square one, tracing the pattern of the divine energy to the cause of the hiatal hernia, etc. Auntie Mary would chant I'o to call in the sound of Lono, grace received in gratitude. What was happening was the receiver's vibration was rising so she could love her husband and heal the relationship.

Harry's Story: Fishing for Tilapia

From the time when I was eight years old till about twelve, my mother, Janet, was a waitress at Coco Palms Resort, Kauai. My father was the assistant manager. He had been there when Elvis filmed *Blue Hawaii* in the fifties. That was when the hotel was at the height of its success. That's why they were making the Elvis film there, because it was the finest resort in Hawaii at the time. It had four hundred rooms.

It was easy catching fish there on the grounds of the resort, which was the former royal residence—a very beautiful spot filled with tradition, power, and beauty. The lagoon had been the fresh-water "icebox" for the Ali'i (royalty). You know that scene in the film where Elvis was married? That's the same lagoon.

So in 1966, when I was quite young, I was fishing for tilapia there one day when Papa Bray came by in a golf cart with resort owner Grace Gustlander. She asked him to come over to Coco Palms frequently to sustain the energy of harmony there on her property. He must have spotted me, for I heard him ask her to stop the cart. I looked up, holding the fishing pole.

He looked at me straight in the eyes. I felt this blessing come to me. Thundering grace.

After that moment of infinity, vertical time, I had reference to kahuna powers. I was conscious of what was happening. I was different afterwards, engaged and affected. I could see things that other people didn't want to talk about.

After that my mother started asking me to fix her feet. "Come over here, Harry, fix my feet for me, honey." She had developed heel spurs being a waitress. To get me to do it, she gave me five dollars each time. That was a lot of money for an eight-year-old boy. And I thought healing was lots of fun as a child. However, even then I also thought it was powerful of me to have this thing I could do that had such an impact.

Soon Auntie Mary wanted her feet fixed, then three or four people, pretty much native Hawaiians. All older women. Auntie Mary can attest to this.

Oh, that lovely woman, Auntie Mary—Rev. Mary, as I always knew her. She was one of the hidden kahunas. She was five foot two and carried 350 pounds. (In the islands it is known that mana is stored in the physical body. Great size, great power.)

She was a minister in Kapai'a, Kauai. She encouraged me to take up the practice of kayaking every day when I was in recovery from law school and academia. The kayaking was a form of meditation practice to bring me into the Pa'a, the now, and out of the Pa'a, at my command.

She said to go out and practice kayaking every day, so for about two years I kayaked. She said that kind of chest and body work discipline would give the power of breath to me. From the kayak, I trained holding the space of vertical time. In the flow over the water, my breath would guide and hold me suspended in no thought—only prayer in action. Breathe and flow, on water, the earth element of emotion. Kayaking gave me Pa'a by shaping my body and mind, so that moving in and out of the state of Pa'a would be an effortless caress of attention to the movement of air in my own body.

Auntie always preferred the rivers of Kauai. "Paddle up and down," she would remind me. "Up for resistance, and down for luxury. Learn to play with the current of the river." It worked. It did take about two years. She never told me in the beginning that the power from the discipline of moving over water would manifest this abundant resonance of humility, tenacity, and penetrating knowingness. For me the kayak brewed the healer's sense of authenticity and sovereignty right into my being.

Auntie Mary had a particular way of counseling. She would open the Bible, to any page, read the story meant just for you, and then she would tell you what was important in it to you. She was famous. Her congregation was fisher folk. They would ask her to bless their boats, businesses, homes, buildings. One of the big roles given to kahunas is to keep the land sacred, to keep its harmony intact.

During this time, I was in KaPaa High School in Kauai, where I was freshman and sophomore class president, then senior student-body president. Then I went to the University of Hawaii, got a B.A. and a masters in communications and mass media, followed by two years of law school. I was twenty-two when I was done with school. That was all I could take. Yah, like they were eating the heart of my flesh. And Sila and I, although we had always known each other, had met.

Preparing to Be a Lomilomi Giver

HARRY: Auntie Mary was teaching me the ways of the healing kahuna by sending me out on the river to kayak. The silence, the water, the trees, the air restored me to my inner silence. In the old way of teaching, a kahuna would accept an apprentice and send him or her out into the rainforest. The apprentice had to learn from the stones. These stones corresponded to every single point on the physical body. There were 365 stones, every bit of the body was covered. The apprentice had to learn the names, the treatment, and the parts of the body inside and out. The stones had power. They were polished basalt from the volcanoes. When the missionaries came, they required all the stones to be dropped into the sea. Cast into the sea.

We still have the secrets even if we don't have all the stones. Remember a monster cannot survive in an environment of gratitude. So whether that monster is an inner unworthiness or a past memory of guilt, harm, or pain, the giver should look into the mind to see where the receiver lives. Emotional maturity is the fortitude to know oneself better. Healers do this, releasing first their own emotional stones, and then they are ripe for helping others bloom. Be free of the emotional stones that show up in your own body first, before you try to help others.

You prepare as the giver even before the receiver comes into the room. You direct your Uhane to tell the Unihipili to activate compassionate disengagement in the Au'makua. You make the four declarations of the Halau for the Lomilomi giver.

When your Uhane, your will, makes the four declarations, your Unihipili, your Low Self, will hear and convey to your Au'makua, your heart self/High Self, to take charge, and all the beings in all the dimensions, the Halau, will hear and share the session from your pu'u wai, heart. With that you cannot go wrong.

Four Declarations of the Halau
for the Lomilomi Giver

1.

My presence in the Halau is a sacred manifestation from me to myself to shower gratitude, growth, and bliss to my whole being and through me to the receiver.

2.

I focus to enter into and to sustain my temple for Lomilomi in the Pu'u wai, the sacred space of the heart. From the heart and through the heart, the essence of my light, my Uhane supports, guides, and graces my touch.

3.

I commit the energy of certainty to the abundance and perfection of my intuition, as I am radiant in the Light of Aloha.

4.

I will my will to compassionate disengagement. I am sustained by Aloha, the breath of God is in our presence.

Teachings on the Four Declarations of the Halau

1. My presence in the Halau is a sacred manifestation from me to myself to shower gratitude, growth, and bliss to my whole being and through me to the receiver.

> I am here in my whole being. From my bliss I extend, shower this bliss to you, the receiver. It is important to me not to use my own energy and will. I use that for entertaining. I am stabilized in my heart, in pu'u wai, who makes the decisions. Bliss for both of us comes from that shower of energy from the Halau.

2. I focus to enter into and to sustain my temple for Lomilomi in the pu'u wai, the sacred space of the heart. From the heart and through the heart, the essence of my light, my Uhane supports, guides, and graces my touch.

> The Uhane is an amorphous movement, not really a noun but more a verb. It is the Spirit of Will in the solar plexus and also radiates from the sacred space in my heart. Uhane, different from psychic energy, is capable of communicating with the receiver in this dimension. I am in intuitive communication with my own Au'makua, High Self, who can communicate with the receiver's Au'makua directly. The Uhane is my integrity and authenticity, a verb integrated in the electricity of the Holy Spirit.

3. I commit the energy of certainty to the abundance and perfection of my intuition, as I am radiant in the Light of Aloha.

> My mind settles and rests; doubt and emotional self-consciousness are put away, shifting out other energies that come from outside by using my heart core by the Uhane. My Uhane is using my heart core to shift out other energies that come from outside. The radiance in the light of Aloha comes from the intelligence of the bottom of the Breath of God in my own end cycle before I receive the next gift of breath. The bottom of the breath

transmits me to other dimensions to the light of Aloha to work on the receiver. The light of Aloha is the intelligence that comes from the Breath of God in our presence. I do not work here into Aloha—Aloha moves through me. I become radiant in the light of the work just as the receiver does.

4. I will my will to compassionate disengagement. I am sustained by Aloha, the Breath of God in our presence.

In other words, as a Lomilomi giver, place your ego, as defined in Western psychological terms, on a big, fat couch where it is comfortable but not part of the session. Let the ego be comfortable, entertained, safe, and not interfering. Let it watch the session, but not think or claim that it does the work. If at the end of a Lomilomi session, you, the giver, are exhausted, you missed the point and let the ego rule. Use your Uhane, the will of spirit , to empower your choices. It is a natural law for the ego to own everything, but the ego's will does not do the healing. So put the ego away comfortable on the couch, then everything goes to the Source for healing.

Questions About the Four Declarations of Halau

Question: How do I will my will?

That's a big question. Number 4, Compassionate Disengagement, sustained by the light of Aloha, is how to will your will. *Will* has two definitions. The American version means the ego empowerment of choice. In Hawaiian, the Unihipili, unconscious will, is the Low Self, representing your body. Uhane is the spirit of will, integrated in authenticity, integrity, and knowing, and grounded in the light of the spirit.

The Unihipili comes into the being's body with the first breath at birth, even though the body is alive in the womb through the mother's breath. At the first Ha-breath, the in and the out, that's the Unihipili arriving. Hawaiian science of healing arrives in the Pa'a, the now, stays in the Pa'a, the now, and knows no other dimension than the Pa'a, the now. The unconscious will is just the representative of your body. That's all it is.

You know you don't beat your heart, grow your hair, digest your food. Actually you don't do very much—Unihipili does it all. Yet the unconscious does not have a past or a future. It has references, memories, but its consciousness is in the absolute present. Unihipili will not let you die. However, Unihipili gives loyalty to Uhane, Spirit of Will, and Au'makua, higher consciousness, so if you choose to die, it will give up.

Unihipili does not go to the other dimension with you. It stays with the body. Unihipili loves the Mother Earth, the planet, so it stays here. Body consciousness stops. Unihipili is not an entity, not a noun, but a series of elements. It creates itself from a list your Au'makua, the High Self, gave it. The Uhane, the emotional body, absorbs whatever consciousness is available at death and that moves to the next dimension. The Uhane, the emotional body disengages from the body and its molecules.

Use this affirmation: "I will my will" or "My Uhane wills my Unihipili" or "I declare my will to compassionate disengagement." Firm direction will help your sessions. The Unihipili wants to engage, to participate.

If you get this one page on the declarations, you get the whole game. And it's simpler than it feels. It's not academic. Certain principles of the will that are a state of being that we can actually declare into our presence.

"I will my will to compassionate disengagement and I am sustained by Aloha." Or to put it another way, take Eden with Adam and Eve. God says you cannot own a creation because if you do, it won't create. You must separate from the creation so it can sustain its identity of itself. This is a critical metaphysical reality.

Question: That's when you get drained, when you don't separate?

Everyone is linked to each other's energies, so they can get well. You have to separate in doing a session. Take pets, for example. Their will rules. They will attach to you and drain your energy and pick up all your illnesses and die sooner from those illnesses. They have will-to-will loyalty. We have heart-to-heart loyalty. In heart-to-heart, no one is anyone's dog. (See more in chapter seven).

Question: So, saying these declarations before a receiver comes for a session can help both giver and receiver?

Life is the energy of intelligence. Raise your energy, your metabolism, and light moves through your body. Because everybody who is in this Halau has been before and will be in the future. Because there is only present and presence. There's no coming and no going.

So when I make these declarations, I invite all beings who share this comfort zone in all dimensions. With that Pu'u wai, you are never going to go wrong. All the resources of the Halau are available to you. Stand up, be bold, and be happy! Ha!

Technique #1: Creating Space

In this technique for Creating Space, you, the giver, direct the force of gratitude from your Uhane to the body of the receiver. The body knows how to take care of the body. When the gratitude is released, it sends signals to the entire body to heal whatever the wounds may be. The body is the superhuman computer that manages all our healing. Remember pain is proof of the memory of emotional stones.

Five quadrants of the body are the focus in Lomilomi for Creating Space: the two hands and the two legs plus the head. These form the star we know from Leonardo da Vinci as the perfect human form. In Lomilomi, the polarity of the star is harmonized.

1. OPENING GRATITUDE POINT: Gently shake the first hand while you and the receiver both practice the Ha Breath (see chapter four). While continuing the deep breathing, place your other hand on the receiver's thymus point in the upper chest just below the collarbone. The thymus switches on and off the various body systems, according to Lomilomi kahuna teaching. As this alternating

energy pulsates, there will be a rush of energy into the chest. And a supreme moment of gratitude may ensue.

2. CRANIOSACRAL TECHNIQUE: Now come around the table so you are standing behind the head of the prone body. This craniosacral technique is known from ancient times to the healing kahunas. Place the fingers gently under the medulla oblongata, cupping them lightly. Pull the head resting in your palms slowly, gradually towards your body. Do not use your strength. Simply lean back slightly with gravity and tenderly bring the head along with you.

3. Next, rotate the head on the brain stem with finesse and gentleness, turning the head from side to side, back and forth, and then in a soft circling motion around the top of the spine.

4. Move the tips of your fingers to lift and stretch underneath the cranial area in a light one-two-three pulsing pattern.

5. Now, move around the table to the receiver's toes. (Resist the temptation to use oil on the feet. Later in the treatment you will smooth warm coconut oil into every nook and cranny.) Confidently grasp each toe in turn, gently pulling each digit, releasing any tension or stiffness in the joints. Now, be generous with the coconut oil, giving special attention to the pressure points and the boney edges around the ankles and sole.

6. Finish the Creating Space technique with similar attention for the hands.

Remember, do not use your muscle strength, use your weight as a lever of gravity with a smile, and relax.

• • •

Harry's Story: Witnessing Healing in Vietnam Vets

Old Hawaiians in the hospital started asking for me. They were calling me. One, Uncle Robert said, "Harry, chant. I cannot die in this vibration. Raise the vibration and chant." Word started getting out. I never picked Leila or Renee or the guy who survived his cancer—they called me.

I never had an issue about charging money. People just threw it at me. The strangers, people not of the Hawaiian culture, mostly Vietnam vets hiding in the forest of lower Puna district, on the Big Island, came by word of mouth. Somehow one heard, came to the back door at night, then others. Now we know they had Post Traumatic Stress Disorder (PTSD), but then there was not yet a psychiatric name for it.

These vets lived in the jungle. They had bought surplus army tents. They were outside the society, growing pot, canning it, and sending it back to the United States. Even *60 Minutes* came and did a TV show on them, how they were living, how crazy-wounded they were. The vets exchanged food stamps for treatments. At the time, they got $140 a month, spent about $40 on food. Back then the food stamps looked a little like currency. They were Hawaii's second currency. You could use them for food, or to get your car fixed, or to buy pigs.

These guys were American rejects. They were reliving Vietnam every night, full of horror at what they had seen—and done. One man had a horrendous amount of energy in his body from the teenager he had killed. I spoke to the ghost of the boy and asked him to let the soldier go.

Now with Iraq, it's happening again. I saw a young man in March going through the same agonies of attached entities, or ghosts of people who died violently. The vets need more than medication and group therapy. Lomilomi, especially the Bone Washing and breathing, helps. The Vietnam vets wouldn't accept massage and coconut oil from a man, but they would allow my laying on of hands, breath work, and prayer to exorcise the demons of death and the war. Often the PTS energy would manifest to the Kahuna's inner sight as pieces of men and boys, women and girls who been blown apart as they died.

Opportunity: Aloha's Forgiveness

*Here's an opportunity, first do it with yourself until you have
anchored and made this technique your own.
Then you can guide others—only then.*

1.

*Close your eyes or leave them open. Take a breath, hold for a
count of four. Continue to be aware, ala, of your breath.*

2.

*Now shut your eyes and look in, where you keep the energy of a
person not yet forgiven. But from a disengaged place,
feel—get the feeling of unforgiveness.*

3.

*Now you move to a new space of your being that holds the name of
a person you have forgiven already. Again with the support of breath,
feel the energy now of the forgiveness. This is* pono, *balance. It is
in this different place, the third place of pono, where the most
healing energy is contained. The pain is stored, waiting for
a catalyst to activate your personal healing energy.
For yourself, for your True Self.*

4.

*Take a breath and release. Take another breath. Drive your attention to
one person who holds for you a thank you for participating in her or
his life with support and Aloha. But for some reason or another, you
avoid, or have avoided, the receiving of that energy of gratitude from
someone who appreciates you. Now, release your attention, notice the
gravity of those Step 1 memories leaving your Paʻa, your now.*

5.

*Then think of a second person. Then a family—or a broken family
or a cluster of humans and animals that are of and like family.
Or another person, or two others. It does not matter. If they are
grateful to you, they are the space in your mind/body that holds
the most grace for healing that is available to you. So think of this,
and breathe, and connect to your unreceived energy of gratitude.*

*That gratitude belongs to you completely; those other negative
feelings do not. And that gratitude is always open to you. So you
can go back in time, be the witness, accept the gratitude, not the
shame, and you will notice the flow of healing. This is not in the
forgiving, but the place of being, one place where what has been
given is gratitude did you did not accept. Unforgiveness/forgive-
ness—move through both/either of them to receiving gratitude.*

*Imagine a bowl of poi that staple food of every Hawaiian meal.
It would sit in the center of the table, at room temperature. The
islands' average yearly temperature is 75 degrees. Naturally a sour
crust would develop around the edges, but the center was the
sweetest. So you learn early to pick from the center of the bowl.
Understand that the rough, tough edges may be hard, but the center,
the healthy center, houses the sweetest, the nourishment. If someone
asks you to take, be not short with yourself. Take a big piece from
the center. Big piece—big charge. Then you will see tears of joy.
Don't go for the crust of unforgiveness; go right to the center of
your being, which is gratitude and its companion forgiveness.*

Sally Ann's Healing Story

When a friend invited me to her home to meet a Hawaiian kahuna, I was fascinated with the ease and flow of how Harry worked. It entranced me. I especially was interested in how he kept focus. I asked him if he could help me. He referred me to somebody else. To me, a professional, his integrity jumped way up. When I heard Harry was going to offer a Lomilomi training course, I took it. First I noticed his kindness, then his connection of Oneness with all life, to the Creator, the wave, the flow of universal energy. And that was all happening at once.

I think Lomilomi chose me, not vice versa. You don't get to turn away from something that's face-to-face with what's meant to be. You don't get to turn away from truth. My heart and mind opened to this experience in Lomilomi; it's not something that's done to you. Lomilomi forces you to move. The energy moves through you like a conduit, and you change.

The energy goes through both of you, the giver and the receiver, settling into something super deep and comfortable, like home. The longer I practice Lomilomi, the more settled it becomes, the connectedness of all things. Sun, trees, ocean, everything that is, moves through you to others, to persons, to animals.

Lomilomi practice is like home, contrary to how society thinks things work. It opens a door into you. We are all healers at our core, if that's your intention. You open the door within and find the universe. I had been trained as a registered nurse, then in counseling, first as a hospice volunteer then a grief counselor. I was especially assigned to sit vigil with families. It was incredible, being part of the personal work people do at the end of life.

After the first Lomilomi class, I bought my massage table right away. I bid on e-bay until I could afford one. The minute it arrived, I wondered what I had done. But Harry says: "The minute you get afraid you're doing the wrong thing, you know you are on the right path. Everything you do expands you."

Now when I go into hospitals, grocery stores, malls, I just consciously raise my vibration using the exercise Harry taught us to do. Consciously breathing with the intent to raise the vibration for all. Then people will raise their own vibrations or leave the area. This simple consciousness protects me from stressful vibrations.

When I am doing Lomilomi, I feel the Halau, the oneness, apparent. The Halau is other healers on the other side, the circle of healers of another realm. The more you do Lomilomi your sense of what's happening in the other body increases. You find their glitches. Also each session, you attune yourself more. Your body takes in more energy. I go up after a treatment. It does not drain me.

I would love to see Lomilomi done in hospices. I had an experience with my own aunt dying. You know, it takes strength to die. It takes energy to die. When we sit with someone trying to die, doing Lomilomi or Laulima, it's so powerful how he or she takes the energy to pass. I could feel with my aunt the sense of peace, a spiritual feeling as our energy levels leveled off. "She was restless before you came in," my cousin said, "Look how peaceful she is now." I knew it was her High Self that drew me to her. At the end I was the only person she recognized. She talked to me about taking her out, getting her hair done. As soon as I would put my hands on her, she would close her eyes, breathing changed, she relaxed. There was love in the room. Her son could feel it too.

Part Two

Temple Lomilomi
Techniques

HO'O MANAMANA—EVERYTHING is a manifestation of divine energy. Yet we each are responsible as conduits of that power, that divine energy for Aloha, the Breath of God in our presence. To Hawaiians, perhaps to Polynesians generally, one person cannot be well alone. It takes many hands working together like a family to produce the desired results. *Ohana* means family. Healing, even survival, takes a family, a community, a whole communion. Lomilomi, specifically *Laulima*, laying on of hands, is a key step for building healthy communities and essential to preserving and restoring planetary wellness.

As we move from the healing of the Whole Earth to working with one receiver at a time, we take the kind step of serving all, because we are all family. Start with where you are and who you know to share the Aloha Spirit. Begin nonverbally simply being the Aloha Spirit, breathing consciously to raise the vibration, then build your practice person by person.

Many healing issues, such as wellness, self-determination, and self-respect, depend on having healthy communities and healthy people who can actively participate in the process leading to empowerment. Harry's objective for sharing the Temple Lomilomi is, therefore, to have family, friends, and neighbors growing community health care that is receiver-centered. Thus Harry continues teaching with practical techniques you will learn for hands-on healing.

Chapter four introduces Technique #2, the Ha Breath. In chapter five you will learn Technique #3, Laulima, a group laying-on-of-hands session. Chapter six includes Technique #4, Bone Washing and releasing cherished wounds.

The Ha Breath: Grace Receiving Gratitude

Harry and I met in Herkimer, New York, to work on the book. We sat in a picnic area near the Herkimer Mines, while Sila took some tools into the mining area. Harry and I studied the ground, turning over gravel, finding Herkimer crystals even near the picnic table. The sun was easy going, we talked about Harry's early experiences leading to his full-time commitment to healing.

Grace and Gratitude

GARNETTE: Would you explain what you mean by "grace receiving gratitude"?

HARRY: Grace is the inalienable right of all beings to receive the light of God, the inalienable source of all healing. From the power of God comes this completely unconditional love, which heals and propels support. Grace is absolutely free. You don't have to do anything to get it. Grace is not something that can be taken away from you, in the Hawaiian point of view. You do have to acknowledge you are human and humans have grace inalienable.

It's really a re-remembering you have grace and thus going back to your authenticity of who you are. When grace appears in the consciousness the natural response is gratitude.

Gratitude is the action linking the grace to us. Grace connects and deepens the channel of gratitude. Hawaiians acknowledge the grace received—it is natural and so evokes gratitude. Alice Mammoser, my colleague in Buffalo, uses the concept similarly. She says, "From Him to me to you to Him."

Naturally. that's all that needs to be healed—the re-remembering of grace, even when people are sick enough to die. Laulima is effective one-on-one, but most effective communally because of the shouting of gratitude that happens energetically. Thus wholeness pushes away any degeneration of disease.

For Hawaiians, two higher vibrations are the easiest sources for healing: (1) Gratitude: communion through gratitude; (2) Laughter: the purest form of communication and communion with God.

GARNETTE: And you breathe more deeply in order to keep on laughing. It's a circle of life, is it not? I've been doing some laughter therapy at our local hospital for cancer patients and staff. When they laugh more, they breathe more, and the stress floats away.

HARRY: The loudest, cleanest, direct communion with the Light of God is joyous laughter of well-being. When you laugh, you cannot think. And that's good for healing.

Harry's Story: Leila's Legacy, Her Teaching

For five months after I withdrew from a life sentence as an attorney, where I experienced law school as eating the flesh of my heart, Auntie Mary sent me out in a single-seater kayak. She made me buy my own, not simply borrow one. I needed my own vehicle.

Auntie Mary sent me to Wailua River, to the rivers Anahola, Wainiha, Kealia, Hanapepe, Kalihiwai, and Hanalei. There are five sacred rivers on Kauai, each representing one of five continents. The Wailua flows in the southeast end of Kauai. This area is extremely fertile. Hawaiians are so accustomed to being surrounded and living in the colors blue and green. The Wailua is deeply blue and intensely green with ferns bowing to the waters. Silence is there.

In this pure silence, only the sounds of the wind, birds, water, and my paddle, I came back to my peace and my authenticity that had been submerged in academia. Law is the path of some, but mine was to be that of my heritage, my lineage, a kahuna. I paddled along the sacred river, room-size ferns overhanging the banks, I thought about my life and my work to come.

The river is sacred. Two rivers join together at the Wailua waterfall that defines the beginning of that Wailua Valley, a whole geography. A culture thrived there in the wettest conditions on earth. With 408 inches of rain a year, it appears to be a swamp. You probably saw it if you went to the movie *Jurassic Park*. Remember the scene where they go to an island? As they go inland and up, there are hundreds of waterfalls. That's not a Hollywood studio set. That's *Waialeale*. And that's where Auntie Mary sent me to ponder my life. This valley was never surrendered to the invading Polynesians or later conquered by King Kamehameha. The kahunas who held this sanctuary sacred would raise the winds by so much spiritual management that it remained a strong hold of independence.

I am going to teach you a mantra. In English: "From Him to me to you to Him. Mother Earth, Father All, I acknowledge you. I splash the wave. I activate the wave now. Come."

On other islands, the surfers may call in the big waves with *Ho'opaipai hele mai kahea*. In the precolonial days this *Au'makua moana a* chant was known to the kahunas on Kauai for initiating healing, calling the waters for the crops, and protecting the islands. This is what Auntie Mary sent me out to do.

It was there Leila found me, some might say idling away the days, savoring the filtered sunlight, shadows, and deep places on the river. Paddling, drifting, becoming one again with the sky, water, and dappled green. The word for fresh water is *wai* in Hawaiian. There's another word, *kai*, for seawater. Water is life's blood to the kahunas, who are masters of the water element. A kahuna is master and friend of the Spirit of Water.

Let's call her Leila. I am not going to tell you her real name. That belongs to her family, her Ohana. Leila was of the native Hawaiian lineage. She and I had, of course, known each other throughout our schools days; every Hawaiian child knew every other one on the island. Auntie Mary had sent her to find me. Leila, who was then nineteen years old, was entangled in a life-challenging diagnosis.

Auntie Mary sent her to me. She had this knowing about Leila that she would soon die—and a knowing about my path. Auntie Mary told Leila she didn't need her Lomilomi—she needed to find me.

You see, Leila also knew she had a few months of life left in her body. It was part of her knowing and her trust in the larger life of the Spirit. She asked me to stay with her often and until the end time. Hang out, be with, walk with her on her dying journey. "Harry, do my feet please, it helps so much with the pain." But mostly Leila wanted a witness, someone who would treasure her story and share it. "It makes it easier," she said, "to relate to my own age group." She loved her family. That's why she was still on the planet. But instinctively she felt she needed someone her age nearby.

Since I had no judgment of her, when I asked her to let her family know she was cooperating, she agreed to take her chemotherapy although she knew she would be dying. She asked me to share this truth—that she knew she was going to die—to share this truth with her, since no one else could or wanted to believe that. I was twenty-six years old.

There was no mourning in her, she revealed, because some months previously she had been near death and saw heaven. Heaven opened up like a golden vision before her wondering eyes. And she was told in the vision she would have another two months to say good-bye out of love for her family. All drugs, the morphine drip, various pain medication, and other interventions were useless.

At the moment I seemed to have the depth she needed. I did a lot of Laulima, laying on of hands. We sat together in silence. We breathed together. She did the Ha Breath when the pain built up. She died exactly two months after she had seen heaven. She received her healing and was ready to leave.

I share Leila's valiant life story now, as she wanted me to, in order that others may face their issues with courage and the truth of the golden vision she saw of heaven. She is living on in the blessing. Telling her story is proof of her having life. She still has life, just without the body.

(GARNETTE'S NOTE: Sila said when Leila died, the family sent a helicopter out about a mile over the ocean to scatter Leila's orchids and plumeria flowers in the water. Some blew back and hit Harry and Sila like a farewell. It was really strange because she and Harry were standing about a mile away on the beach.)

Technique #2: Ha Breath

Harry often begins a Lomilomi session with seemingly simple instructions to the receiver to be aware of the breath while lying there on the table. "Close your eyes, listen to your breathing. Adjust your breath so you are comfortable with watching yourself breathe. Breathe in through the nose, hold it to the bottom of your lungs. Breathe out through the mouth with a strong *HA*. Keep your attention on the breath."

• • •

Breath as Medicine

HARRY: The real conduit of healing, the core, is in using breath as a medicine. Breathwork is primarily grace receiving gratitude.

The giver's attitude is that of breathing with the receiver. Mano, the shark, is a perfect angel because of the quality of piercing decisiveness. The shark is protected in Hawaii's ocean; no man can kill a shark without incurring legal punishment. Mano gives the energy of receiving piercing decisiveness as an intention. If a receiver can welcome piercing decisiveness here, that's all it takes. For attention is the shape of gravity in the mind.

Piercing decisiveness is the tool you use to receive grace to heal. This means you become like a shark with a receiver, healing in faith. Forget images of the shark as fearsome. Instead understand the gift the shark brings by its being. When the shark comes to you, you learn focus. You learn to focus the mind with piercing decisiveness—in a playful, Hawaiian, laid-back way. You are swimming in the great blue ocean of God, and you are determined to keep your mind one-pointedly focused on what you want to heal.

You focus your attention with breathwork. You pay attention with breath to the receiver. Through your affirmation and coaching, the receiver creates the connection to grace. Breathwork is the cord the kahuna uses to reconnect the receiver with grace.

Breath—deep, powerful breath beginning in the diaphragm, at the solar plexus, the space between the lungs and stomach—is where the power to heal comes through. The connection to grace comes through the diaphragm. The diaphragm is the basket of emotion where the Unihipili (Low Self, your friendly unconscious) can create a will with the Uhane to heal then empower the Au'makua, your High Self. That's what healing is. And that's where you get your facilitation.

The Unihipili activates a language between your Au'makua, your authentic self, and your body. This is the recognition of the presence of grace. Naturally comes the gratitude thereafter.

So the breath begins and gathers power in the diaphragm, echoes as it moves through the heart, then into the throat where it becomes a spoken chant.

So you will hear the kahuna chant *A ki mele ahua a pu'u* when a session begins. *A ki mele ahua a pu'u*: "I connect with you in the song of my heart, the master of my soul." *A ki mele ahua a pu'u*: "I connect with you in the song of my heart, the master of my soul."

This is the way emotional language, the language that heals, moves. The diaphragm is like the drum. The diaphragm is a vacuum. Breath activates the emotional language, beats it like the drum. Then this real breath movement flows with emotion when the kahuna gives voice to the healing. The chant is the en-chant-ment.

GARNETTE: Harry, that makes me think of the song "Some Enchanting Evening." We know the stranger you meet across the crowded room is, in fact, your own unconscious, your own Unihipili projected out onto a person. It's the song itself, the breath involved in the singing that flows the emotional language out to your own trifold self. Then the healing occurs and love fills the air?

HARRY: Yes, there is more to that song than meets the eye. It gets the breath flowing from the solar plexus, like island music, activating the heart, then singing forth from the throat. And the result: grace revealing gratitude received. That's what you experienced, was it not?

GARNETTE: Many times. When my partner used to put his hand on my heart, I felt like a galaxy burst open and streamed out light. That light was powerful, emotional. During my first Lomilomi session, after he died, I then recognized what that feeling had been: gratitude. I reexperienced blessed, blessed gratitude. I felt like I was the queen of grace. That's why I wanted to write this book with you. "Some Enchanted Evening" was our song, as it was for so many others who knew our spiritual teacher.

HARRY: The Ha Breath is a powerful healing tool. Givers are recommended to stay with the breath during the session. The healing will occur. That's why I can say a Temple Lomilomi session is two to three minutes of light, of gratitude, and all the rest is dancing with the body. You felt like through the points of resistance, like you could have danced all night, right?

GARNETTE: I'm still dancing, Harry. What is it about the gratitude wave release that makes us feel so great?

HARRY: Lomilomi. Lomilomi raises the vibration. It frees the cause of the pain, frees the pain from the crystallized emotions held in the body. And when the Ohana, family or community, comes together to lay on hands in Laulima, the release can be cosmic, such as you experienced.

An Anonymous Healing Story

I met Harry Jim in the summer. A psychotherapist I went to for marriage counseling recommended him to me. She said he could help me in working though and releasing emotions. As I respected her, I went. Although I really had not known what Lomilomi was about, I had some experience with alternative therapies in the past. I continued to choose Lomilomi breathwork because of the results I was getting. My progress was unmistakable.

The work I did under Harry's skillful guidance was mostly Lomilomi Ha breathwork. I had appointments with Harry for one to one-and-one-half hours on approximately a weekly basis for twenty or more sessions. I think I was unusual in seeking so many sessions, but I found them so profoundly helpful and different each time.

A typical session would involve discussions with Harry about issues since our last meeting (usually related to my marital relationship). He was always very present as a listener, and I appreciated his comments from emotional and spiritual perspectives.

After our discussion I would lie down on the massage table, and we would begin the Ha Breath with him coaching me in a deep-breathing pattern. It was work to keep that breath going, but at some point I would notice a shift into an altered state. Each session seemed to have a different feeling or theme. There were times of physical releasing of anger or sadness and times of great peace and bliss.

I was always aware of what was going on and felt safe that Harry was there, connected to what was happening. Each session was valuable and sacred, whether it was physical release or travel in an altered state. I was so grateful to Harry for guiding me though my healing work. He was endlessly patient, compassionate, and professional. He helped me to recognize my own strengths. The sessions were a vehicle for deep connectedness with Spirit, and the breath is a powerful vehicle.

Tana's Healing Story

(Authors' note: Tana, an artist, supplied this written account. For authenticity, we have retained her distinctive asterisks and lowercased words.)

* * at my first session with harry, he did breathwork with me. he guided my breathing (full, deep, fairly rapid breaths through both my nose and mouth) until i felt intense vibration in my eyes and mouth. i was surprised by the strong buzzing sensation . . . it was very strange, and so strong that my mouth felt uncontrollably pursed. harry said that the areas where i felt the vibration corresponded to issues i was currently dealing with. he suggested that i felt it in my eyes because i was resisting "seeing the truth," and in my mouth because i was resisting "speaking my truth."

harry worked on pressure points on my feet as i continued breathing, then he moved up to my head. as he worked on my head, i started to feel a ball of heat form in my stomach . . . . i have since referred to this as the "freaky heat ball." the heat became more intense, and it started to kinda freak me out, so i mentioned it to harry. he said, "yeah, i see it . . . we're gonna move it on out." and as he worked on me, and as i continued the breathing, the freaky heat ball moved up to my chest, and as it moved up through my body, it got hotter. then it was in my throat, and really hot, and that REALLY freaked me out. then it moved up through my face, on out the top of my head!

harry was busy throughout this bizarre occurrence, but i could not tell you what he was doing . . . . i was way too distracted by the freaky heat ball! *(um, pardon me, mr. kahuna, but you neglected to warn me about the freaky heat ball . . . .)* i teased harry about it this past weekend. i said to my practice partner, with harry there listening, "watch out for that guy . . . he'll pull a freaky heat ball out through your head when your not expecting it!" harry, of course, sat there and giggled.

* * one of the most important lessons harry has to offer is that of nonjudgement. this continues to be a very valuable lesson to me personally. i once asked harry how one could avoid unhealthy energetic connections to others (i.e, how one could interact emotionally with others without risking an energy drain). he said that such a thing is not possible if one holds no judgement. in other words, if i am judging someone, i will form an unhealthy energetic connection with them, but if i have no judgement, this does not happen. harry said that he is able to do the work he does without being energetically compromised or depleted, because he holds no judgement towards his clients. to carry this lesson further, one is not capable of true compassion if one is holding judgement.

harry's nonjudgmental and fully compassionate approach is one of the main qualities that make him such an effective healer. i feel entirely safe exposing any and every part of my bruised and twisted psyche to him . . . . i can be completely vulnerable, and at the same time feel completely protected. (and how many people are there for *any* of us to be able to express *that* level of vulnerability with?) he creates this entirely safe, loving, healing atmosphere . . . that is his greatest magic. though i must admit, all his bells-and-whistles-voodoo is pretty great too!

** at harry's most recent workshop, someone humorously used the term "harry's girl's" to refer to her local group of fellow students. while it was just a joke, it made me think of the importance of *not* giving harry guru status. while he may be deserving of this billing, labeling him as such would clash with one of his most important teachings . . . that we *all* have equal access to the divine! while it would be so easy to view harry as a guru (i mean, c'mon, he looks like the laughing buddha himself!), i feel that to do so would actually be disrespectful to his teachings. harry constantly stresses that we are *each* equally valid expressions of God, and that we do not need him, or any other intermediary, to connect with the divine.

to give an example of what i mean . . .

at my first meeting with harry, he said to me something like, 'i see you as the greatness that you are,' and he is teaching me to, likewise, see *everyone* i meet as the "greatness that they are." at this past weekend's workshop, after a three-hour lau lima marathon, i looked around the room and thought, "my god . . . i'm in a room full of buddhas! and i'm a buddha too!"

CHAPTER FIVE

Laulima:
Laying on of Hands

Harry's Story: Laulima

When I was four, Tutu, my great-grandmother, was sick. So my mother and I visited her house. Just before we left, everybody gathered around Tutu's bed and placed their hands on her. You don't learn Laulima. It was never explained. Everybody expected you just to do it.

Others call it laying on of hands. It's a worldwide tradition. In Hawaii, it's ancient. *Lau* means "pulling in" and *lima* means "hands" (sometimes it means "thumbs"). So *Laulima* means pooling of hands. *Ohana Laulima* means the family pools hands together for family. That's what I was doing with my mother when we visited the sick. It was just natural. Just be. That's Laulima. There may have been prayer—probably was, as prayer is also natural. So there's a prayer to begin.

Everyone born on the planet knows Laulima. That's how you know who you are. Laying on of hands is not related to ordination or training but to understanding your own authenticity. Laulima is a giving time. It's grace receiving gratitude.

What happens after fifteen minutes of Laulima is an emotional safety net anchors people so they never have to fall into lower vibrations. If they fall vibrationally, unwellness occurs. Laulima, grace receiving gratitude, sustains wholeness.

And yes, Laulima is usually about someone who is facing a health issue. The family gathers to get them better by walking them into the full vibration of love. It's simple. You just do nothing, you just be.

The Many Meanings of Laulima

Laulima is another of the multilayered words an observant person will see as abundantly in Hawaii as fresh pineapples. It's a word that has legs. One layer of Laulima, that of the community pooling together, is the name for a collaborative program supporting reflection and problem-based learning through the use of Laulima software.

On the Big Island, in Puna, near Harry's home, there is a community-based garden project named Laulima, "many hands working together like a family." Ohana Laulima is the name of a model community; a sustainable farm on Maui; a taro festival; a health-care program on drug awareness; a Mac users' group; and a canoe club and luxury facility for weddings, retreats, and meetings. There's a volunteer trail association called Laulima at Summit (*Laulima o Haleakala*), the national park in Kula.

GARNETTE: *Laulima*, some Web sites say, means "managing softly through cooperation."

HARRY: Yes, *Laulima* has, like *Aloha*, multiple layers of meaning. I told you Hawaiian language is like that, amorphous. In Temple Lomilomi, we are focusing on the spiritual level, although these projects have spirituality as their core. Why? Because caring for the earth, like the trail association does, is holy work. As is the drug awareness, the community garden, even the software. You know that at the basis of all action is the Oneness of the Creator and the Creator's love and care for creation.

GARNETTE: I found a Web site with a beautiful saying about Laulima:

Bright rays of light would only shine
If each beaming ray should slowly combine
Such rays would create a path for you
A path in which you shall choose
Like burning sparkling flames of fire
Working together would fulfill your desire

And there are several churches using the concept of Laulima listed on the Web as well. In a way the World Wide Web is an electronic Laulima, is it not, Harry?

HARRY: You can say that, Garnette, if you like.

GARNETTE: So by working together, like a loving family, that's Laulima?

HARRY: Yes, and it is also Aloha. Laulima is the practice of the Aloha Spirit where we all have a spiritual connection with each other—and with our land. By working together, everybody experiences Aloha. Raising the vibration by the generosity of Aloha, practicing the Presence of the Breath of God with us, a group laying hands on someone with a health issue is Laulima. You see how at the center of the spiritual meaning of Hawaiian words, all is only one.

Laulima is delicious. It's energy work in the least complicated form. Laulima is quite miraculous, for it is actually the Divine Light's intention for people to feel better.

Remember, in Laulima, God is present. When two or more people gather together, God is there. Laulima is not your energy, but God's.

GARNETTE: Harry, how does one keep from the busyness of doing? That's a trap for people who think that they are healers. They drain their own energy and effort into the other person from the desire to do a healing.

HARRY: Instead of "doing the healing," healers must become the witness to God's healing energy in their hands and God's healing energy in the people next to them. And God's energy in the person on the table rising up to join with the Ohana Laulima. You are simply a communication tool of the Presence of God's breath. You are Aloha then.

Healers may experience a feeling in their hands like puffy clouds. Or you feel a pulse beating in the person as he or she comes into harmony with the pulse in your hands.

Not everyone doing Laulima may agree on whether the energy they feel is hot or cold. Many people have an investment in what they have previously learned, but it's the same vibratory experience. Because from the group comes the common expression of God's Light prevailing.

Technique #3: Laulima

 1.The group comes together with a person wanting to receive Laulima. The person may be lying on a massage table, in bed, or, if needed, in a wheelchair—somewhere they can easily be comfortable.

2. Someone may or may not offer an opening prayer.

3. Members of the group sit down around the table and put their hands on the person, closing eyes to focus inwardly on the hands.

4. There is silence. About ten minutes pass.

5. The person may tell what they experienced. Tears may come.

6. Group members share what they experienced with no judgment.

• • •

The Experience of Laulima

HARRY: A group may be any size, from two or three to four or five and so forth. The person remains fully dressed, as in all of Temple Lomilomi techniques. Each member may, or may not, agree on the experience. But all will probably note that the energy in the person on the table moved. There may well be a significant change physiologically, but the real change will be the real presence of emotional safety and faith manifested by the entire group, by both the person receiving and those giving grace-receiving gratitude.

The receiver may well feel lightness feeling like a levitation. That's a common experience reported to me. Then they may report pulsing, warmth, awe, love. The common thread running through all comments I've heard is sacredness, although everybody's experience of energy differently expressed.

Music playing softly in the background is not necessary. Silence is good. The time does not matter. It could be fifteen minutes, could be five. Longer than fifteen is not necessary. However, when I do Laulima in my practice with a receiver, I may have silence for an hour, if that's what's called for. But with a group, even a few minutes can be very powerful for the elevation of energy. There is potency in more than one set of hands.

GARNETTE: What about Reiki? And how do you explain the popularity of Reiki these days? Even in some hospitals?

HARRY: Reiki is welcomed in Laulima, but not emphasized. Reiki is one on one. The givers are trained specifically. Laulima everybody can do. Reiki is so popular because it works. It gives the giver permission to touch with spiritual intention. In Laulima there's less effort than other modalities. Laulima is free and is simply the laying on of hands with the spiritual intention that the Breath of God's presence be with us. Receivers may be joyous and feel buoyant with energy. The United States is ripe for the spiritual touch way.

Auntie Mary , who was a recognized minister, was absolutely doing Laulima. She would be called to families. I remember her coming in, opening her Hawaiian translation of the Bible to a particular verse that would apply to the situation, lead a prayer to Jesus Christ, and join the family in Laulima. Auntie Mary saw no difference between the Hawaiian's beliefs and the Christian.

"There is no god in the Hawaiian realm not in the light of Jesus Christ," she taught me. Hawaiians readily understood what the missionaries were saying about Jesus. They understood completely "love your neighbor." What they didn't and couldn't get was the devil piece of Christianity. To Hawaiians evil is dumb and entirely predictable. They couldn't get why the Christian missionaries thought Satan was so intelligent, especially since Jesus died for everyone. Who did that leave out? No one. And who did he leave in charge? Our Selves—the true, High Selves of us.

So, yah, the old Hawaiians loved Jesus when the missionaries talked about "be not afraid" and Jesus, the good shepherd, the wise elder, the loving son of God. Weren't all loved by the presence of God? For sure. So Auntie Mary did Laulima and prayed to Jesus. And people were healed.

In modern Hawaii, Japanese Buddhists married Christians— a lot of people from diverse religions married. But it is not about their religion if someone is in pain or sick. Then the person is open to healing.

GARNETTE: Is that why people get sick? Is the pain a cry for community?

HARRY: In some cases, yes. But many others, especially people who have experienced serious cancer and recovered, view their journey as creating opportunities for emotional evolution. They might even say the disease recovery was miniscule compared to what they had accomplished, how they emotionally matured and changed compared to what else they have been through. Cancer survivors know the peace that comes out from their own drive for authenticity. Many times even persons dying come close to Spirit through the process of dying. They become emotionally evolved in preparation of being closer to God. I am not alone in knowing this; anyone who works with the dying always knows that.

GARNETTE: Yes, that's what I am saying in my previous book, *On Angel's Eve*. Fear not dying for God is love welcoming your loved one home.

Hawaii and Dark Kahunas

GARNETTE: When people hear the word kahuna, some think of sorcery?

HARRY: In Hawaii, we practice the Gospel of Inclusion. Just look at all the peoples who have been drawn to the islands. Dark kahunas exist. It's a question of fear or fear not.

Let me tell you about some of my research. I went through the medical records of Queens Medical Center, records from 1903 to 1910 and even into the 1920s. Many death certificates of newborn and neonatal babies cite the cause of death as "kahuna prayer." Even if the child died of whooping cough or influenza, the doctors wrote "kahuna." This led to the laws that drove both light and dark kahunas underground.

In some cases, the cause was kahuna prayer, that's true. A lower vibrational kahuna, or dark kahuna, could change the destiny of a person by prayer.

GARNETTE: Can you really call something that's so negatively used prayer?

HARRY: It's more like command than prayer as you think of it. Since you understand the paradigm of Unihipili, Uhane, and Au'makua we spoke of earlier, you sense what I am going to tell you. The electrical assets that all kahunas use as techniques can identify and separate energies. The dark kahuna can cause the unconscious, the Unihipili or low consciousness, to pull away from the person, and then they take control of the person's low consciousness. Say someone was dying; the sorcerer would call to that energy and train it to do his bidding. We call those low energies trapped by these dark kahunas "dogs." For they would train the dog to do their bidding by consistently feeding it, just like a pet we might have. This dog used to be the will of another human being. One reason the dark one could do this is there is so much fear sometimes in dying.

This is different from Voodoo, which attracts earthbound spirits to do the giver's bidding.

The separated Unihipili would be fed with attention, with energy. If the sorcerer was really, really bad, he could have a pack of dogs.

GARNETTE: This gives some people the creeps.

HARRY: I have to address this in my workshops because there are always questions. People want answers. People fear low vibrations, but there's nothing to fear as long as people keep their vibrations high. Fear has a resonance people can feel, even if it comes from the past. Lomilomi is about letting go of the past, and thus the fear. There is so much fear today.

GARNETTE: By politicians, marketing, TV ads, and cable news shows?

HARRY: No, the ads are directed to the Unihipili in people. The dark kahuna uses a weak, low consciousness that has already left the body-mind-spirit continuum. Garnette, there are more enlightened kahunas than just the one or two dark ones left. These dark magicians are not only Polynesians, but also from certain tribes in Africa and China—even Christian-professing magicians. The original information was seeded throughout the planet in twelve tribes, not just the Polynesians. The loudest, cleanest, direct communion with the light of God is joyous laughter of well-being. As I said earlier, when you laugh you cannot think. And that's good for healing. There are and always have been two practices, light and dark. Always the practice of light is more powerful than the practice of dark. Kahuna, minister, person, everyday people have two choices. To take the dark path of power over other being or the Light path of serving other beings.

In the verb of *kahuna* there is access to both potentials. A chance to make a choice. A chance to expand in service or to close down in power over others. It's the lightness of service versus the darkness of power. Light vanquishes darkness by raising vibrations to light with breath. The choice rests in the heart, the Uhane, while it manifests in the ego. In my courses, I teach how to sterilize the darkness of power. I learned this from the white kahuna, a great man.

The answer to nullifying the urge for power is in the phrase "Am I enough?" If the answer is a definite yes, then the path is service. If the answer is even the slightest vibration of "No, I am not" then that's the path of power. Of trying, trying, trying to be enough, to have enough power.

GARNETTE: Oh, like the famous saying of a billionaire when asked how much money was enough. He replied: "Just a little more."

HARRY: Yes. Let's sweep away the whole idea of "not enough." Each person's Uhane has the power to be enough. The first step is to serve yourself. This is very important. Take care of yourself. Say "I am enough." This gives you the path of service.

GARNETTE: Is this self-confidence? The large Self of God?

HARRY: "I am enough" means "I am connected to God." Not enough means not connected to God. It's that simple. It's Hawaiian. When you have just a mild belief, one person is not enough. But when doing Laulima with five or six people, that's enough to disengage the belief of needing more power.

"Power" here means power over other people's energy. And that's what, to the Hawaiians, is the premise of evil. And I want our readers to recognize, that there are a lot, lot, lot fewer dark kahunas (DKs) than ever before. Part of the reason is the genocide of our people. But the biggest reason is that the energy it takes a DK to feed his dogs is not available any more. Why? Because the prevalence of Christianity has made dogs less available. And when I say Christ consciousness, I mean Buddha, YHWH (the unpronounceable Hebrew word), Krishna, and the Divine Mother as well as Jesus Christ, and Lono and Kane in Hawaiian. The supreme light spreads dominance over the whole being. When a being is in the light consciousness, no DK can reach her or him. With the world of pure light enveloping them each with a cloak of protection, there are fewer people willing to believe and give their spirit to a DK. For a drug abuser, there's no will there to give anyway, so they are at big risk.

GARNETTE: So that's why the dominance of the colonizers troubles Hawaiians. It's power over other rather than serving the needs of the sacred land and her people by a democratic process. What about that story of the dog in Max Freeman Long's book *How to Make Miracles*?

HARRY: That's a most entertaining chapter. Long's colleague is on the side of a volcano. A boy is dying, and the colleague sees with his third eye "dogs" coming at the boy. So Long's friend uses his will without prayer to free the boy. Since the dark kahuna who'd sent the dogs underestimated the man's will, the DK's power boomeranged and went back to destroy the DK himself. This is a true story I heard before I read it in Long.

Do you remember Papa Wai? He's gone on now. He spent two hours a day with his guides. When he was called to do Laulima, he would find out if the person had someone else's will attached, affecting the person, even before he gave herbs. Papa Wai spoke loudly and often about relationship. He inquired about any ill feelings in the family, in relationships. He would clear the person of those ill feelings (dogs again), and they would be healed.

This is pretty heavy about the sorcerers, but we must have some meat in the book. There are some wrong books about Hawaiian kahunas. The number of DKs are small—always were—but sensational. Now if people know in their hearts and will say, "I am enough," they will be free of dark thought-forms. Remember life is about service to all, not power over others. And laugh—keep on laughing.

Annie's Healing Story

Thank you, Harry! Thank you. Thank you! I use Lomilomi all the time in my massage practice here in Hawaii. It is like a spiritual essence that I was initiated into by him—Harry. He looked into my eyes, and I couldn't stop crying. Then I loved the dinner and lei making. I needed that sense of family. It was deeply touching to a lonely, disconnected person like me. I was deeply moved. I would love to repeat the course just to share four more magical days with Harry and the others at Yoga Oasis (the Hawaiian educational facility and retreat center in Lower Puna, on the Big Island where Harry and Sila hold biennial workshops).

On my way to the class, my neck and head started to ache. It got progressively worse until the third day. At the Laulima, laying on of hands with a group, I had to run to the bathroom to vomit. The others in the circle didn't even notice. When I told the group, one person thanked me for vomiting his garbage. Another said I had got the feeling from her. After that I began to feel better. I felt like a lot of garbage left me forever! I met two wonderful women there who mothered me the whole time—which I desperately needed. And Harry assigned me to his teenage friend that I could bond with. I needed that healing as well. Woman to woman-girl. I think he knew that. It was very powerful. Thank you, Harry. Aloha Nui.

An Anonymous Story:
Teaching Energy for Physical Fitness Trainers

I teach in the physical-education department at a community college, where I teach fitness as energy. Even though I talk about it in terms of the chemical name for energy, I'm still planting a subtle seed in case students eventually find themselves opening up to other, more subtle forms of energy, such as the chakra system, meridians, and qigong. For me, it's about making the concept of energy simple, understandable, and usable, and I begin in the simplest and most easily measurable of terms—physical energy. It's this way that I can make the power of energy approachable.

Well, I have mostly activity classes, so, typically, after brief instruction in the building of energy systems, emphasizing the chemical system of choice (aerobic, strength, power, etc.), the students spend the rest of the semester mastering the activity of choice (walking, jogging, weight training, etc.) But this semester, a new class was added to my schedule—a strength and conditioning class as part of a new personal-training certificate program at the college. This class has a weekly lecture component to it, and, feeling the need for something new to teach, I accepted the assignment. Shortly after the weekend intensive, I found myself implementing Huna philosophy in life, as well as fitness-training principles, as it supports fitness as energy. For example, shortly after the weekend intensive, I found myself expounding on "90 percent entertainment, 10 percent fitness" (see chapter eight) to motivate clients to continue to seek personal trainers' services. And just this past weekend, I talked about "attention"—as in, if you want to feed your business, feed your clients with attention and watch your business grow.

Even though Lomilomi has nothing to do with strength and conditioning training, I have found myself incorporating the Hawaiian philosophies into the lecture portion of my class. I don't plan these things, but I can't hold them back when they want to come forth. And it simply supports the subject matter and seems to make the material more personal, better applicable, and less like "work." Even though they don't call it a "WORKout" for nothing, it's more like inspiring them to health and fitness instead of making it a chore, work, or, even worse, punishment.

I think the reason the philosophy of Lomilomi comes so effortlessly and lends itself to fitness training is because Lomilomi itself is action. It's because of that Lomilomi being a verb thing. It's action. Health is action! Health is vitality (energy) in motion; the action of living life. And the better your energy, the better the quality of your life. Also, because I needed that intensive like I needed the air. Lomilomi lives in me and breathes in me—and when the opportunity comes up to share Lomilomi, I just can't help but do that with all my heart.

CHAPTER SIX

Bone Washing:
Releasing Cherished Wounds

Before clock time began, the Hawaiian healer saw the perios-teum, the skin of the human bone, as the cache where memory of physical movement, memory of painful emotions, and memory of abuse lurk. These memories store up one after another like rocks that eventually become mountains. But those memories can also be brought to the surface and released through hands on healing called Bone Washing like the lava disgorging from volcanoes over millions of years to form rocky outcrops. Volcanoes took eons upon eons to clear the pathways from the center of the Earth before Hawaii became a Paradise. Although we don't have that long, in one life, we can bring forth the hot rocks of our hurts and wounds to create a paradise of health in our own bodies.

But like the early Hawaiians, who could not sit by watching the debris from the volcanoes clog up their taro fields, we cannot let the debris of our feelings clog up our body's pathways as it's released. It was the dharma of the kahunas to keep the water of the taro fields flowing clear. They would *kal'ai* to let the nourishing water flow into the fields. In the realm of taro growing, "to kal'ai" means to clear and repair the streams so waters flow and run free through the various pathways of the taro patch. As the paths clear, the nutritional balance of the field is consistently available for growing that staple food of Hawaii. Obviously, clearing the path creates the state of abundance and health.

In the same way, Temple Lomilomi kahunas kal'ai the stagnant muscle tissue and scrub the bones of the receiver. Discard the picture of the healer taking out the bones and washing them in a pot. No, that's not what Bone Washing means. In Bone Washing, the giver places his or her fingers on the receiver's body and, moving the fingers between the muscles around the bones, directs energy to clear out the energy of the remembered wounds. Bone Washing cleanses the fascia, the muscle tissue. The Lomilomi kahuna gently wash away the strain and pain of the energetic weight of the person's interior world.

Try it on yourself. Press a sore spot on your body now and see if you can get in gentle touch with the memory underneath it. If it's a small grievance, you may be able to release it with your Ha Breath and the assistance of the Aloha light. If touching the spot uncovers a memory you've been protecting yourself from, find a Lomilomi giver trained by Harry, and gently, patiently, you will be assisted in clearing it.

Technique #4: Bone Washing

 After the Lomilomi receiver has Created Space and coached the giver in the Ha Breath, the next part of the session is Bone Washing.

1. The receiver should lie comfortably and fully dressed on the table.

2. Starting closest to the heart, at the left shoulder where the channel may need washing, the giver places the fingers of both hands between the muscles to the periosteum, the skin of the bone. Focusing only on the breath, the giver's fingers will move slowly outward toward each extremity, applying pressure using a light touch of the fingers. The fingers will move in rhythmic semicircles, establishing an even, rhythmic pattern of one-two-three, one-two-three.

3. After the left arm has been completely Ka'lai'ed all the way to the receiver's fingertips, the giver then moves around the table to the right arm and repeats the Ka'lai.

4. After the arms are completely washed, the giver washes each leg in turn, starting at the hip and moving down to the feet.

5. The giver then moves behind the table to Ka'lai the head, called Po.

You do not need to "help" the process along.

• • •

Benefits of Bone Washing

HARRY: Bone Washing can be done through out the entire body but especially on the arms, legs, and head. The body's emotions will then accelerate. A zest comes, stagnated emotions move. All kinds of emotions are corralled and moved, freeing the receiver for the zest of life. The Bone Washing modality can empower profound changes in the use of the body.

Bone Washing is done carefully, foregoing any pressure for focus. Focus is the golden key in Lomilomi. By focus the healer's intention manifests. Focus is best done with the receiver and the giver in thoughtful communion with the intent. Focus is the imagined idea of what to do. As the intent is to clean the blockages on the bone, the blocks will leave the area and become agreeable to the intent of direction. As the healer you will intend that the energy or base substance will stop being a logjam and flow on eventually out of the body itself.

This is the kind of work that evolves the receiver doing the Ha Breath.

For most receivers, light pressure is just right. It's not about heavy pressure moving all the muscles aside. But for some receivers, you may use heavy. Your wisdom, your Au'makua, will guide you. Once you move the energy, and you can feel it move with practice, rechannel the stagnant energy into the Earth. Use a gentle one, two, three touch.

GARNETTE: Mother Earth takes that energy and recycles it for her own purposes.

HARRY: Yes.

You must be prepared that nobody leaves Bone Washing with a complete flow from head to foot. Just like daylight cannot stop from shining, the energy of the heart cannot stop moving from Bone Washing. The energy once unblocked will continue to flow. It just may take clock time.

GARNETTE: Is this the Hawaiian way of describing kundalini, the understanding of the Hindus that energy is light moving up the spine radiating throughout the body-mind-spirit? The chakras and their accompanying organs are blocked by lifetimes of emotional and karmic wounds, which keep kundalini from flowing from the base of the spine to the crown chakra in a circular flow.

HARRY: No, the Hawaiians know from ancient times that energy moves in the body like an inverted infinity symbol, the figure eight. *Kal'ai* means to clear old, stagnant energy and to clear cherished wounds. Bone Washing relieves ailments: any diagnosis of stagnation, repetitive muscle pain, weeping but not able to cry, anger, poverty, slavery, abuse of all kinds, genocide, war.

Harry's Stories: Kal'ai Bone Washing

1. Seven years ago, a sixteen-year-old came in. He had had a soccer injury years before and with the use of other therapies, he had seemingly recovered. He was playing again. But his gluteus maximus hurt. In other words, he had a pain in the butt. (Maybe he was a pain in the butt as well; we don't know or judge that.) As soon as he walked in, my Au'makua knew he needed Bone Washing. I put him on the table face down and focused on his hip, working down the outside of the leg to the smallest toe to kal'ai the pain out through the foot. He was confused, as he had not associated the butt pain with the soccer incident. But as soon as the energy left the tip of the toe, he stood up and told me about the soccer injury.

There was no decision to be made about treatment. The pain was locked in; it needed a path. There was no need for a meditative state or recalling or reliving the injury first. The healing just happened by the kalʻai, clearing the path. The effect was the result of our resolve and focus.

We didn't have to figure out his belief system. Or why he had the pain. All that can come after, if the receiver wants it. Or beforehand as a fanfare to the energy being released. The energy tells you why. I am asked all the time about why the energy was blocked. Let's focus on the fact that it's not blocked now. And it won't return.

2. Doing 'Po'—clearing the suture muscles on the head: A forty-six-year-old Hawaiian man came into the office on the Big Island, two weeks after he'd had a small stroke. It was small, but a stroke nonetheless. He came after he got out of the hospital because his MD sent him, having done all he could do. The man also had Bell's palsy. To kalʻai this long-term problem was my immediate focus.

He was on the table face up. I focused on his neck, doing Po, up the side of the neck into the face, and hit his emotional charge area. He had a stuck energy of fear there. He must have all of a sudden noticed this energy of fear and had had the stroke. His body and energy system suddenly noticed it (meaning it became too big or intense to ignore), so the fear erupted physically in the form of a stroke. Stroke is a common manifestation of fearing the future. I continued up the skull over the right eye through the suture muscles that hold the cranial plates together. And the path cleared. His symptoms were gone.

When he told the MD, the doctor said, "It was not the kahuna, it must have been the Coumadin" (a blood thinner). The Hawaiian just smiled and nodded, said OK. He called me after he left the doctor's office, laughing. He hadn't been on Coumadin, the blood thinner. He wasn't taking it.

3. The matriarch of a large clan came to see me in Puna. She came for a treatment but never mentioned her son's demise from using crystal meth. She told me about her middle-back pain.

I asked her to lie face up (for back pain!) on the massage table. The sliding doors of the room were open to the coolness of the banana trees and a trade wind. It was Hawaii at its best, that day. I focused and began on her breastbone, up to the collarbone, down her left arm to the ring finger, kal'ai-ing a path so that all that anguish would leave. She couldn't stop shaking at first. Her pain was caused by the absolute shock and disapproval, the *real* humiliation of his drug use. The shock, disapproval, and humiliation actually belonged to her son, but she had taken these emotions on herself.

She was owning his pain, and it needed to find a way out. We already talked about how a negative force can jump on a survivor. She loved him, but he had to get off her. He needed a way out of her, and she needed to get back her life as the respected leader of her Ohana.

Lomilomi: So Different, it's Pa'a

Temple Lomilomi is so different from other modalities. Other methods say go right there and do this no matter what the issue. In Temple Lomilomi, erase that, erase expectations; disengage analyzing; pull way from history and references and then you will be empowered by the now, Pa'a. As I remarked earlier, if you gave up all your belief systems that you came to this planet with, there would only be a little spark of light above the chair.

> *Pa'a. You are in the Pa'a when you stand on a surfboard,*
> *only when you infuse life into your garden;*
> *only when you gather and sew a lei of healing flowers;*
> *only when you ride a horse—*
> *with all of yourself and all of your attention.*
> *You can call it the now. It's the Pa'a.*

Proof of the Pa'a is alignment with all that is. Pa'a is the evidence of now because you are enormously strengthened. And that strength is displayed in your actions.

Congestion of power in the receiver is exchanged for the energy of change. Thought is the first thing to disengage from. Analyzing. Referencing the past. It's a big concept—the Heisenberg—that the observer changes the activity. Apply that to Bone Washing, and you find that the less you do, the more your energy can do. Less is more, for the more comes from the receiver's spirit, his or her Au'makua from the point of Pa'a, the now. Then the charge is really discharged.

And when that blocked energy is discharged, the clearing goes seven generations back and seven generations forward. Spirit goes into the past and the future and heals. The healing will go out into infinity. It will go into your family's genetic memory, into your great-great-grandmothers' lives.

And it will not go in English either. It will go in the language of emotion. The multidimensional language is emotion. And the greatest of all emotions is laughter. If you want to raise a vibration, to vivify the vibration, laugh and chant, "I-O-E-I-O" (long a, long e, long o). The I'o is the Hawaiian hawk, a word of all vowels. It's the Hawaiian *Mawri Tonga* (one of the Hawaiian deities that is a verb) whose reality cuts transference.

Say, "I love me" and/or "I am enough"—that really cuts transference. Your imagination is accurate, so say, "I am enough."

You will find while doing traditional Temple Lomilomi, that Bone Washing is fun to witness. You expand the vibration, build the vibration. When the totally unselfish hands lay hands on for healing, you are becoming planetary. This is the medicine of the future. When connecting with someone, you will want to acknowledge that something bigger than the two of you together is present and actually doing the healing. And then, when you feel that, you know what Temple Lomilomi is and can mean for this Earth, our island home. Prayer is the core of Hawaiian massage, because Lomilomi is prayer in action. Lomilomi is prayer that extends into activity. Not prayer of supplication or pleading or by a ritual voice, but a prayer of communication giving union.

Jo-Anne's Healing Story

I first met Harry Jim and first experienced Lomilomi six months ago. I first began writing this testimony three months ago after completing a four-day Lomilomi workshop with Harry. Writing tonight, I can truly say that Lomilomi and Harry have impacted my being and my life, precipitating change in ways and to a degree that I could never have imagined.

Very simply stated, I have found "myself." I know that I am now integral. I know peace, and I know joy in my life and in myself. At forty-eight, I have found peace with myself, with my past, with my purpose, my future. I am inspired by a new sense of connection with others and life. Lomilomi and Harry have proven to be vehicles of profound liberation, revelation, and transformation for me.

I'm someone who's searched always. Sneaking into my parents' bedroom, I poured over my father's psychology textbooks at age ten. Driven by teenage and existential angst, I engaged in passionate philosophical and esoteric conversations with my grandmother. During my twenties and thirties, I dabbled in so many practices, but ever so briefly. I then resigned myself to the belief I'd never find peace and understanding, or a sense of community of spirit with others. My choice of profession is surely a reflection of my fascination and drive for evolution, meaning, and connection. I remember always the quest, the drive, the need to understand myself and to find peace in my being, with my being. And the drive to know my place in the world.

Even my coming to experience Lomilomi and meet Harry is to me amazing! I was, six months ago, deeply anguished with a sense of being stuck in my life. I came to realize that this anguish echoed the sense of "no way out" or dead-endedness that I'd experienced when in past abusive relationships. With this realization, I knew it was time to return to therapy, to tend to my soul and effect a change. A beloved friend suggested a therapist whose name I'd often heard. The first session was stunning for her piercing insight. As we closed, she suggested I call Harry Jim, simply explaining he is a Hawaiian who practices Lomilomi. With absolute trust and a desperate heart, I made an appointment.

I've met with Harry for probably eight to ten sessions of Lomilomi. From the first session, a profound and vital dynamic of change was unleashed in me. I know now it was precipitated by my courage and willingness to sound the depths of my heart and soul, trusting in and converging with Harry's incredible insight, skill, and ability to create a holding space in Lomilomi, a sacred space in which incredible repair, awakening, and growth would occur.

From the first session, my experience was profound. Stunning. Radical change and movement were initiated. Synchronicity began to manifest immediately! Within days I met ex- and current colleagues who'd been working or studying with Harry for one to two years. I'd never known. I'd never heard his name. I'd never heard of Lomilomi. Suddenly, Lomilomi and Harry Jim were everywhere around me! I was finding an unknown network of which I was becoming a part.

So inspiring was the experience of Lomilomi and the liberation that I was experiencing in my mind and heart that after several sessions I decided to attend a four-day Lomilomi workshop with Harry. I wanted more. I wanted to learn to do Lomilomi and to offer to others the potential for the transformative, loving experience I was enjoying.

I began the workshop in tears of emotional insight and release. I completed the course truly knowing that, as Harry says, "I am enough." I learned experientially that weekend that I am, in who I am and what I bring, enough. I realized that all of the self-doubt and judgment was false. I am by virtue of my essence and presence, enough. I am, beyond my body, my intellect, my manners, my sociability, perfect and absolutely all I need be. I left the workshop thrilled by the experience of receiving and especially of doing Lomilomi, changed by the insights into myself, the acknowledgement and experience of my essential, personal strength, and by the communion with the others.

I am humbled and amazed at how I have emerged into myself in the past months. While I continued erratically with therapy, I focused intensely on Lomilomi sessions for a period of several months. I believe each and both have been important to the changes I have experienced and effected. I believe one has complemented the other. However, I have experienced the capacity for transformation by way of the body and the space for healing created by Lomilomi. No mind, no intellect—just integral, essential being.

I've changed inside. My life outside has also radically changed. Lomilomi has facilitated my breaking out of the excruciating dead end I was experiencing six months ago. Immediately following the workshop, I interviewed for a new professional position. I began my new job in April. It's a new, vibrant, exciting and enriching position and opportunity. Just as I feel I've come into myself, I feel this position is a reflection of coming into my just reality, one of respect and self-respect, ease and opportunity. It's also allowed for a radical change of schedule, and freeing of time, energy, and opportunity.

I am so happy with my life and with my self. Lomilomi has truly facilitated my release from past troubles and a coming into myself, into self-acceptance and stepping fully into my life. Practicing Lomilomi offers me the experience of being fully present with myself and another, of knowing "I am enough." It has allowed me the amazingly beautiful experience of creating a sacred, safe, transformative healing space with another. It's what I love to do and to experience. It's where my heart and soul soar and touch the depths of my being at once.

Laine's Healing Story

I met the work of Harry actually when I started the workshop. I heard about Lomilomi in massage therapy school, then stumbled on his Web site. I decided the Lomilomi workshop was perfect for me, and I drove from Pittsburgh to Fredonia, New York, for it. I felt like I had a dose of laughing gas. A feeling of light intoxication and much needed relaxation. Like conscious unconsciousness.

I choose Lomilomi for many reasons. I believe it is a tool for me to add to the toolbelt of my body-work practices. Also, in Pittsburgh not many people know of Lomilomi. I would like to show them that, like me, they can become part of this bubble, this

Halau, a family of energy. I learned about vibrations and energy. It was a real experience I will never forget and want to share with others.

Lomilomi is illuminating, warm, and felt like Hawaiian sunset. It's an hour-and-half vacation to the islands. Everyone should experience the benefits of Lomilomi.

Part Three

Living Aloha

IN PART THREE, HARRY EXPANDS on generosity, hospitality, and groundedness. At his workshops, and often slipped into people's hands intuitively, Harry gives out a printed card with the Hawaiian Rules. While they are funny and perhaps provide people with an "Aha" moment, he means these guidelines to be taken seriously, especially since so many of his friends, students, and receivers are dealing with manifesting abundance, coming free of the ties that keep so many from full and radiant enjoyment of the Aloha Spirit.

In chapter seven, Harry talks about money and manifesting abundance, as well as its opposite, the debris that stops the flow. Its main focus is on the cherished wounds and tantrums that keep abundance from flowing. For in the Hawaiian understanding, a tantrum is defined as when your Unihipili and Uhane recognize and protest that power is being taken from them. Harry regularly leads groups to his Hawaii. In chapter eight, you can experience the atmosphere of Harry's Hawaiian workshops with a transcript of one morning's activities. He answers questions that participants have in the moment.

Chapter nine is a varied and powerful collection of healing events that Temple Lomilomi students, receivers, and Harry's colleagues—medical doctors, social workers, healers, chiropractors, and psychotherapists—have willingly supplied to further understanding Harry's role, persona, and work. You will especially enjoy the final story from an eleven-year-old cellist. We call these Aloha stories of healing.

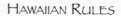

HAWAIIAN RULES

Never judge a day by the weather.

The best things in life aren't things.

Tell the truth—there's less to remember.

Speak softly and wear a loud shirt.

Goals are deceptive. The unaimed arrow never misses.

He who dies with the most toys still dies.

Age is relative. When you are over the hill, you pick up speed.

There are two ways to be rich—make more or desire less.

Beauty is internal—looks mean nothing.

No rain, no rainbows.

Say "I love me," and you'll always have plenty.

CHAPTER SEVEN

The Path to Manifesting Life Abundance

Givers who are starting a Lomilomi practice often have questions about the funding and what to charge. Harry's own sessions are modestly priced. Here's the Aloha spirit of generosity in action. Harry talks not of charging, but instead about creating abundance:

Creating abundance is about manifesting and about connecting. What is the difference between prosperity and abundance? For me, prosperity guarantees you can buy a mango. Abundance witnesses the mango tree in full fruit. Abundance is about moving your vibration. Prosperity is what you earn. Abundance already is. Once the giver's channels are clear, abundance becomes the natural state of a rich life.

People have always just thrown money at me. From the time I was eight years old and my mother tossed me five dollars to soothe her waitress-tired feet. Money flows through the cleared pathways, just as blocked energy flows by ka'lai, Bone Washing, and life-giving water flows through the channels to nourish the taro. It's the same energy pathway for abundance.

The flow is always there. The process was the same in Old Hawaii as it is in the modern world. Human experiences and especially tantrums, often in the teenage years but can continue unless cleared, create the blocks. And continued tantrums block the flow.

There is something about cherishing a wound that defines a person. Cherishing the wound may seem to make meaning out of the horrible. These cherished wounds have their roots in the first restricting ideas you were given when you came onto the planet. Often parents can't bear the beauty of a child, so they become aloof or abusive. Or you may have been abandoned or scolded. We carry these wounds through childhood and into adulthood. Lomilomi can help people deal with and release such pain.

People often lose their power. With Lomilomi, we can see the progressive pattern to this power loss. When people lose their power or give up their power for any reason, two initial premises are operating in them. One is an inability to identify their cherished wound because it's buried so deep in the psyche. And the second is the inability to identify what's buried beneath as a tantrum. Become aware of the problem and you solve it. It's as simple as that.

First understand what is the cherished wound. It comes from the parents' negative ego projecting onto the newborn. This is not the parents' fault, just as the parents' wounds are not the fault of their own parents. That survival-motivation belief system—such thinking as "distance is safe," "silence is not punishment," "what's mine is mine and what's yours is mine," and many other false ego beliefs—is imprinted on the behavior of the young one. The wound is cherished, the wound is protected, because it's the only known love, but it is love sourced from fear.

The cherished wound in early years comes from brutal parents, aloof and distant parents, interrogating parents, or sexually abusive parents. Of course those of us with what would be considered loving parents can also develop cherished wounds. The tantrum is a trance state that prevents our full attention to Pa'a, the now. It's the energy leak created by fear, the belief of not enough. The receivers either have to recognize those elements to make the Lomilomi process flow or the giver will stay in pain from the stagnation. There are some identifiable icons—maybe receivers recognize that their dad was aloof, cold, torturing like the Inquisition, or felt sorry for himself, and that the vital juiciness and brilliance of their life forces have been challenged and contained by psychological chastity belts. The key to unlocking those chastity belts is the light of Forgiveness. Then the power starts to flow easily. The Hawaiian forgiveness process is the kahuna and the person together dismantling and recomposing the belief system that prevents flow, abundance, prosperity in its richest sense. Sometimes receivers will say, "Open my arms (see the Creating Space technique, on pages 50–51), I missed that the first time." This is because they have an idea about forgiveness, that it's patronizing someone else, or fake, or old hat.

The Light of Forgiveness

GARNETTE: How do you initiate forgiveness when the mind is filled with misinformation about it?

HARRY: I source the vibration of the first and second chakras. I source the mana from the Unihipili to the Uhane to the Au'makua, the High Self, to generate prosperity and abundance. It's the same technique we use to generate healing. We ka'lai, straighten out the channel, clean out the muck, using the source of their personal energy. Dismantling belief systems is the work of the kahuna, so the taro can grow and nourish the person. Every person who had a diagnosis of cancer and was healed had to shift belief systems. They let go of cherished wounds and disempowering tantrums from adolescence. Belief systems shift with every healing experience.

GARNETTE: But what if the tantrum is forgotten, buried deep? What if a person is not in touch with their belief system that is making them sick or hurt?

HARRY: Yah, people do have unknown hooks that make abundance flow away from them. So many people have financial hooks. Yet when we are born, we automatically have abundance. Parents may say, "You showed up, now it's more work for me," and that becomes a cherished wound of guilt that the person holds. If the growing-up process locks down a person, the healer has to guide them to unlock and give up the barriers. With Temple Lomilomi, whether it's done by unleashing the Gratitude Point, Bone Washing, Ha Breaths, craniosacral work, or shoulder pulling (see Creating Space), at some point the history is going to be unveiled. That's when the remembering comes forth so you can know. When a person brings to light the memories, the healing occurs.

GARNETTE: What's the difference between who the receiver is and what the receiver wants? And who the receiver will be and what the receiver gets?

HARRY: Space. Creating Space is the process called manifesting abundance. Most every receiver that comes wants that jewel. Creating substance and space between cherished wounds and tantrums is the balance of energy, effort, work, and faith.

The only thing suspended between lack and space is the havingness of unforgiveness, holding on to unforgiveness.

GARNETTE: Absolutely not to blame the victim.

HARRY: Far from it. The hurt prevents the receiver from sharing his or her power, but it started as a safety lock. Once the receiver has created space, the emotional wounds leave. And the receiver cannot heal on one level without effecting and healing other levels within.

Then once they've remembered, when the mind pulls the pieces together, people on the table say: "You know, I've always felt that, but I haven't thought that." You see, there are two kinds of wholeness. One is religion, which is about running away from sin, from the outside. The other is spirituality, which is "been there, done that" and is inside. It's like the joke: to a religious man, hell is something you spend your life avoiding; to the spiritual man hell is somewhere you've been, something you've done, and now you're moving on from.

Of course. Hell is a consciousness discovered in the search for power. Those who rely on Spirit rather than seeking power, to them hell does not exist.

GARNETTE: Harry, could you clarify something?

HARRY: Sure. What is it?

GARNETTE: It seems that your touchstone is your inner knowing, that you have these profound metaphysical, even spiritual, experiences that are interwoven into your being. They are so a part of you that you do not even question why this or that happened or happens. You just say, "Yah, that happens."

HARRY: When I pray, it is not a passive process, but an activity. I live each moment of a session in prayer. Prayer is intergrated, interwoven in my Uhane so deeply by my culture that silent, interior prayer occurs naturally during a session. I recommend my students practice prayer, their own prayers to the God of their understanding. Actually, session is a prayer.

GARNETTE: To be in a state of constant prayer is to be in alignment, awareness, and responding to the greater environment—to be conscious that you are conscious. Thus good manifests from prayer.

HARRY: Yes. Kahunas from the beginning live teaching to move through pu'le, prayer. That's the *aha* awareness from the definition of Aloha (see chapter two). My whole experience with the kayak was to generate that *aha*. Motherhood gives you the same thing—awareness, that awareness that says, "You cannot scare me, I have children."

GARNETTE: You're joking, but I know that experience.

HARRY: That's what I mean when I talk about living in the Pa'a, the now. Not that I am chanting our old sacred words while I am also talking to you, or driving, or giving a treatment, but the ability to respond totally, without judgment. You have an inner knowing that you trust that one thing or another is the right thing to do. By right thing, I mean the righteous thing, the dharmic thing—love in action—that comes from listening to the body right in front of you. The receiver's body tells me what needs to be done; it always speaks its own truth.

GARNETTE: How do givers put love in action?

HARRY: They can honor everything, especially themselves. Know that you are linked to everything and everybody that exists. I was never told to pray. All I have to do is listen.

A lot of people think that the Divine Source is somewhere "up there," but for me, the Divine is all around me. The only way I can be at peace is when I stay connected, not separating myself from what is always around me. Hawaiians cooperate with what surrounds them, ask for help when they need it, and give help back in return. This is the Lokahi of Aloha (see chapter two), working in unity.

Harry's Story

Like everybody I've had times in my life that were tough, really tough. Markers. The death of Harry Uhane Ekau Jim (my name-sake) was this for me.

Grandpa Harry was having a fabulous 69th year. His neighbor friend came over that auspicious November morning needing help moving an old ice box and replacing it with a new refrigerator that had a compartment for freezing. They got the old one out, and the new refrigerator in, but it was more physically straining than they realized. Their work done, and after the costmary share of coffee and toast, Grandpa stood from the chair and lightly staggered, and just before he left the threshold of his neighbor's kitchen doorway, turned and said, "If you ever need me, just call." He took a step in the direction of his home and dropped. His heart stopped.

He died on Kauai at 11:05 am. I was on Oahu at the University of Hawaii School of Law. Mind set in the middle of a midterm written exam on federal civil tort procedures. I looked at the clock at precisely 11:05. A torrent ripple of grief rolled like storm waves out from my gut into my heart, then exploded through my chest. My mind was in a fog. I closed the incomplete test and turned it in, went back to the dorm, and began packing for home.

The wailing in my chest was overwhelming. For a couple of hours I sat on my bed with my packed bag. I knew that Grandpa Harry had died, but only my body and Au'makua knew. My mind would be told later, after I recovered from the waves of shock. At three that afternoon, my mom phoned, crying, saying there was a sad truth to share. "Your Grandpa is in spirit." She said a ticket was at the airport for me on Oahu, and that I was to fly home to Kauai that eve. My Dad and Ohana needed all of us together.

I know there was a reason for this life experience. I left law school and returned to Kauai. Years passed, and my Path was joined with my wife Sila. I had been doing healing work part-time and, like most young people in the Kauai Island economy, working second jobs in the evenings as wait help at the hotels. I had a bad fall on New Year's Eve at the resort, working a big party. I could not report to work because of my back pain, and so I lost the job. Tests showed a fractured lumbar.

I felt I was moving through a tunnel filled with dark, sticky tar. My family tells me that I would sit and stare at nothing for hours and then get furious at them if they tried to get me to move. All I did was sleep, and it was not a restful sleep. My dreams were nightmares, intense.

When I wasn't sleeping, I was staring at nothing. I was angry. My wife and children saw me as demanding, critical, impossible to please, when I had not been like that ever before. I withdrew further and further back into misery. I ended up staying in bed all day, unable to work.

At first everyone thought I was just in a funk. But as the weeks went by, Sila became worried about me. She called my parents. She called the Ohana, family.

When they came to the house, they knew right away that I was being sad over Grandpa's death. Years had passed, but it was evident the work of releasing the grief of the loss was not complete. As soon as I saw my parents, I began to weep and weep huge tears. Auntie Mary came, prayed over me, then told the family to take me to a medical doctor.

I was diagnosed as depressed from untreated sciatic pain. The physician prescribed a six-month course of pain and antidepressant medications. The protocol included physical therapy as well as Cortisone injections around the spine. Aunty Mary commanded that I swim often in shallow but open ocean. I complied with both the physician and the Kahuna. It was weeks before I was able to regain my personal stability and clean perspective. The pain, both physical and emotional, had lost its grip. I never returned to that depressive state again.

Looking back at that period of time, I realize I was going through what St. John of the Cross called "the dark night of the soul." Earth-based religions know the growth that comes from hitting bottom. It was an initiation, but I wouldn't wish it on anyone. It did force a major change in my life where I gained the courage and fortitude to do what I needed to do in life. To become a Temple Lomilomi Kumu: Teacher.

I come from a long lineage of healers, on both sides of the family. My hours of darkness forced me to flow through that path here on Earth. I had not wanted to follow the footprints of the other healers in the family. I wanted to escape what had been laid out for me. Those Kahuna were older men and women when they engaged with their healing work. Papa Bray started at fifty-two. He did not have to hold the two staffs of being a father and being a healer at the same time.

After I finally accepted my destiny as a healer and provider of spirit wisdom from my past lineage, the channels were fully open. Then I became relentless, tenacious about both Ohana and Lomilomi. I felt present, available to be entertained by the adventure, and I explored an array of healing modalities. A key part of my training was working with Auntie Margaret Machado and Ohana for years. I first met her in early summer 1982 on the Big Island. Her school sits in front of a tiny cove at Kee'i beach, about four miles from Pu'hoonua, in south Kona. She was in her seventies at the time and had had a full healing schedule since she was in her teens. She had three children, grown. She and her husband Dan shared three houses—the school, the office, and a private residence further up the South Kona Mountains. She used the beach house in Kee'i for Lomilomi. People from all walks of Hawaii life waited in the garage on folding chairs until she called them upstairs. Up there was a living room with a mat and sheet in the middle of the floor. She just bent down on the floor and worked. She had beds and massage tables on the porch. People were treated on various surfaces, depending on circumstances.

At our first connection she greeted me with a hug and kiss and said, "Sit you down, I'm going to read what is in your being." With her eyes shut, she scanned from my toes to the top of my head, and here, heart open, Auntie grasped the energy of my being. She told me "You are to do Lomilomi teaching." With grace and respect she weaved the story of her childhood mentor explaining how her uncle taught her the ways of healing through witnessing.

She disclosed her memories of the Manoi and Kaimikaua lineages that I came from. She discerned that I had received the early childhood blessings, but reminded me that the real hard work was the training. I would be well served to walk the cleared path of our lineage, she whispered. "It is completely engaging for you to do the work of teaching and healing. It is in the blueprint of your body. You already decided this like me, before you showed up this time."

"My job" she enjoyed proclaiming, "is to work you hard!" That she did. For years we shared the healing work of many people. We also shared teaching people from all over the world the basics of Lomilomi.

Auntie Margaret really liked feasting on Hawaiian food with her husband and me. I fully enjoyed those meals too, so while the others would prepare other food, she and I would have local avocados ripe from the trees, fresh steamed fish, dried meat, coconut stir fry with green and yellow onions. For dessert, we enjoyed rice pudding and sautéed banana in butter. We became good friends, laughing buddies.

Auntie Margaret offered a ten-day program called saltwater cleansing. It cleans the mucous membrane on the walls of the colon. Auntie Margaret and I did this together with several apprentices, learning the process, simple as it was, over and over again, always building on our knowledge from experience. She would prescribe Lomi Lomilomi treatments to me for people who were on the ten-day cleansing program, using this traditional fast/cleanse approach to heal organs and psychologically manifested negative behavior patterns ranging from smoking to recurring poverty. She required people receiving the cleanse to have steam baths twice a day and Lomi Lomilomi once a day. Also long walks near the ocean at Kee'i beach. She gave this ten-day regime to no more than twenty people at a time, and it truly cured their ailments. They would leave happy, well, and grateful.

She made me practice shifting physically and emotionally toxic thought patterns and toxic physical contamination from the receiver melodically. I would take people through what she termed "molting" from the inside out. She advocated constantly the old Hawaiian practice of stopping at dusk to proclaim forgiveness to all transgressions and transgressors of the day and receive the energy of grace from all the grateful people you served since the sun rose that morning.

I have had many teachers whose stories are worth retelling. But none, including Auntie Mary and Auntie Margaret, gave me the education that the many thousands of clients I've encountered in healing treatments over the last three-plus decades have given to me. There is much more of the Divine's Light to witness. Vast is the future.

An Anonymous Healing Story

My wife, a massage therapist, took some classes from Harry and convinced me to give a session with him a shot. My first visit with Harry was an hour-long session in the early winter. Harry warned me before starting that the first session tended to have profound effects—little did I know how right he would be.

For many years, I had been having chronic leg pain, which I attributed to my weight and tough workouts, and no massage therapy or stretching seemed to make it better. He started working on my legs, and for the most part it felt similar to a deep-tissue massage. But as he kept working, it developed a different feel, much like the tingle you get when a foot falls asleep. Then at one point, he was working on a spot on my calf he said was a major energy block. When it finally released, it felt like my foot had shot off and blood was gushing out (not painful, just a sensation). Harry said huge amounts of built-up energy were flooding the room, so much so he had to open the window. (Harry notes: The difference was breathing. Breath generated from the inside. I really just pushed the breath until I got his vibration so high that the fear of taking a deep breath dissipated. He had been breathing shallow for years, resisting that grief that he released in a deep breath.)

When the session was done, I was light-headed, had to walk slowly to maintain my balance, and waited over an hour before I felt comfortable driving again. Since then I visit Harry every six months or so, and I have not had any pain in my legs. He's also helped with my neck and back pain as well.

CHAPTER EIGHT

Lessons from the Hawaiian Workshop

Frequently Harry returns home to Hawaii to see his islands and his hot ponds, to feel the gentle rains, to relish the sun and tropical breezes. He is called back, as so many are, to his roots by his Ohana (family), his Aina (home islands), and the clients he has helped in Hawaii. One year, he gave a February workshop in Fredonia, New York, then flew to Hawaii the next day to give a four-day workshop for the Lomilomi body workers (givers) he had previously trained and for receivers he had previously helped.

The following are lessons and discussions from that workshop, transcribed by Karl Lindstrom of Yoga Oasis. They have been edited for clarity.

Harry's Introduction

The first word for the whole course is the word *ineffable*. Ineffable means an idea or an activity that is not communicable in human language—something beyond the verbal, something amorphous. The experience for most of you for the whole four days will be ineffable. It will be hard to express what you have learned other than through your hands. That is just the way it's going to be.

Miscellaneous Comments by Harry During Introductions

- *Become a healer to heal your own self.*

- *On the table there is no difference between giver and receiver.*

- *The energy of healing can rejuvenate you.*

- *As soon as your soul knows connection with yourself, you can offer body work as opposed to massage.*

- *Not all sessions are body work; some are massage, but, as you learn more about yourself, the more you become capable of holding the space for the person in front of you, and the more the body work becomes Lomilomi.*

- *Hawaiians say that all knowledge is never in one school.*

- *This is a school that teaches more than technique. You can choose to swim as shallow as necessary or to swim deep as necessary. It's all in that river, it's all in that force.*

Before we get into that we are going to spend a lot of good time with each other, as you enter into the Halau. And we will do that before lunch, by creating the declarations (see chapter three).

How You Learn Lomilomi in the Hawaiian Style

This is one of the first cultural differences I want to bring to the table. It's basically four words: "Be quiet and listen." In Hawaiian style, you don't get techniques, pathways—you get "Do you see?" until you get so quiet that you can actually see and feel. When you work with anyone else, they are just showing you a technique. Hawaiian style is allowing you the bravery of a deeper breath; you go to that second level of body work. Our Hawaiian way is saying, "You will eventually get there, I don't have to show you," and if you cannot get there, then you don't belong doing this. Because if you cannot get into that space, you won't survive, because that means you don't have the space to hold that depth. What normally happens is that, if you keep trying, your passion will hook you into the river that's under there. Your passion will hook into that force, and it will drive you in.

This method sounds simple—you do the work, and the wisdom will come. The only thing wrong though with this method is as we get farther away from the Hawaiian culture, there are seeds that are missing—and those very seeds are what I try to present. I do know that if you are called—and what I mean by calling is that if you are sitting in the health-food store when someone says "take this class" and you show up—then you are ready for the seed. You have been being quiet, paying attention, and listening. And so that's valid.

The other seed of our culture is, in Hawaiian, the concept of "No say, do!" That's a big piece in Hawaiian culture: "No say, do!" "Don't just talk about it, do it." Does that make sense? "No say, do!" Empty talking is only a thing; doing is the action, the completion of the action.

Yet there is phenomenal power in your language, phenomenal power in words. When you speak a word, any word, it then has a right to fulfill, to actually express and manifest once you say it.

Hawaiians are never the kind of people to present an expression of how you *must* do things. It's the same when you go fishing with an elder. My dad taught me how to throw net. He didn't say, "Take one third and one third and put it on your shoulder. No, he just said, "Sit there . . . get comfortable, watch me." You know, that's it.

I said, "Father, can I have the net?"

Father said, "Wait, when you are six. Keep watching."

By the time it got to my time, I was like doing "one third, one third. . . ." Because the "sit down and listen," it works. It works for that culture. It doesn't work so well in the transition to the American culture. That's OK. But the "sit down and listen" is still the main rule for dipping into that place. You sit down and listen to your body, because it's reflecting what's happening to their body, and you hold that space. That's what we are going to learn a lot about: holding that space.

Creating Space

The first section is about Creating Space, and you won't find it in any other workshop, for it's the way I learned from older people who create the space for the person to sit comfortably. And it may seem obvious initially. But Creating Space is wherever, whatever depth you want to go with it. So that's why in many classes that you take, there is always: "Lomi 1, Lomi 2, Lomi 3." If you notice, other people who have taken the class will get just as much as the people who are taking it for the first time. Because it frees you to swim as deep as you need to. OK? Trust that. But also, take hold of the force and let it take you. Because you are in a safe environment here and now for the next four days. Because what I want you to leave with is the power to decide . . . "this person needs me to swim deep, this person needs me to get rid of the headache," and have freedom to do both, and receive from the giving. Yep, it's about us.

It's important for you to recognize that while you may not see the whole mango tree full of mangoes, it's because you are only standing on one side. The mango tree keeps going!

If there is any language that clearly describes when that realization happens when someone says: "Oh, my God! There is such a thing as 'world impact.'" Because you made those people feel really good for a long time. Far past the body work. Their mind changed permanently. That's what we want to do—change the mind so that of course they are going to seek out more body work, eat better food, get more exercise, and get healthier and be healthier, and receive gratitude, which is really big—we are going to get to that. So even years later, they still send you gratitude, believe it or not.

Opportunities Given to You in the Space of the Halau

1. *Your belief system will change.*

How many people get that? That after this class your belief system will change, and that after you give a good session, that the person's belief system changes. And the wholeness of Temple Lomilomi is about restructuring the belief system. That's really what it's about. Because the temporary state, it's just a portal, so that those things can come in and out as we choose. Does everybody get that?

2. *You will acquire the skill of shape-shifting energy, in the body and moving in and out of the body.*

Shape-shifting energy is a skill. Not the same but similar to pounding the nail in with a hammer—you have to learn how to do that. You'll do that with the first lesson this afternoon, which is called Creating Space. There will be energy in somebody's torso, and you will shape it and shift it out of the body. So, shape-shifting I know has had a different meaning. In this course it means being able to understand energy and direct it and move it away, simply by Creating Space within the torso. So that is the first thing. You will acquire the skill of shape-shifting energy in the body and moving it out of the body.

3. *Your comfort zone will expand.*

How many understand that the only way your comfort zone expands is when you are uncomfortable? Strain, pain, stress, expansion is stretching. Emotional pain more than physical pain, but pain is a big signal that expansion is occurring. And generally, not always, your comfort zone's expansion is what is required to go deep. For example, "I'm comfortable with this craziness in front of me." Because it's temporary, and so we get past that. And so you will see that. That the craziness isn't always so much in the receiver, but the giver has to have a little craziness that has to expand too. We are tapping that same source. So your comfort zone will expand: you will be comfortable with more. Your belief system will shift; your comfort zone will expand.

4. Your emotional body will evolve to share voice.

How many of you are aware that you have an emotional body? That there is kind of an energetic presence within your own physical body? In Hawaiian science it's the emotional body that leads to the other dimension. The will sets at earth, because it is of earth, and the actual substance of your body stays at earth. It's only the emotional body that moves towards the higher dimensions.

Now some systems call that "Spirit." Right? However, it's an integrative piece of the Spirit, the emotional body. And emotional evolution is the intention of life. Emotional evolution is the intention—in other words, the only thing you take away from the workshop is the emotional ability to be mature enough to hold that space. Because out of emotional evolution comes the idea that you know yourself better.

When Sylvie, a Lomilomi body worker who Harry trained, worked on a couple from Akron, New York, they knew themselves better. They knew the joy they had more than they knew it before the treatment. And that is what echoed all the way to Buffalo. Their ability to know themselves better through the emotional expansion and maturity.

Does that make sense? Is that our goal? That is the major opportunity. Because you can have healing even with people who then die later. Healing is emotional expansion and maturity. Healing is not limited to the definition of rejuvenation. That aspect of healing is incidental and coincidental to the process of emotional evolution. That comes only as a component.

5. You will be able to shape the space connecting the body to the healing window.

OK, there is an actual time in the treatment that seems to converge upon the receiver and the giver, for that single moment, when there is healing. How many have experienced that on your table? That is where we want to go to, right? Where that time actually converges. So we do that by saying: Healing in the Hawaiian way is 99 percent entertainment, 1 percent God. So if you had an hour and a half and you entertained the receiver with body work and for that one second, the two of you experienced God's presence, that one second is where the healing was, because time stopped in Pa'a, the now.

OK, take a breath and laugh at that because it's going to come from a place that there is a reality to that. Ninety-nine percent entertainment, 1 percent God. And your skills to entertain are what you have brought with you to the portal, to the Halau. One percent God, one moment that it all transcends. That's the kick. So that is what that statement number five identifies, the healing window.

That 1 percent, where they just connect, will happen, given the space of all this freedom between the receiver and the giver. And the direction of all this freedom, and all that is going on. It happens. Because there is an operative rule that came even before the Bible came to this land called Hawaii, an operative rule that came before the Christians landed. And that operative rule is "wherever two shall be, I shall show up." "Wherever there are two in my name"—my name being Light—"I shall show up." So it is in the transcendence of witness, witness, witness, that Light shows up. I know it's Christian, but it's also Buddhist. And it's Hawaiian!

6. *You will grasp your capacity to reverse the polarity paradigm of your self-trust.*

I am going to read that again. You will grasp your capacity to reverse the polarity paradigm of your self-trust. OK, now, take a breath and go, "Hu-ah."

In other ways of teaching Lomilomi, you always experience this idea of when the receiver's session is over they will give you acknowledgement. They are going to give you communication that says that you have done a good job. When you go to work for someone and they pay you, you always get this experience of giving trust outside and receiving validation from someone else's

WHAT IS ENTERTAINMENT?

Now I am going to spend a little time on what entertainment is, because we think entertainment is laughter and joy. But I want to point out that a block away from my house, about a mile away from my house, is an eighteen-plex, meaning eighteen movie screens. As you are on the freeway, on the road, you can look at the list of all eighteen movies playing, because there is a huge sign that they change accordingly. So anything that's in America is playing right there. And for a year I have passed that sign, and I looked at it as I passed it, and that's America's most formal entertainment form, which is movies, right? There is always a horror—always a horror. There is always some pet show—some dogs and cats. Sometimes a cartoon cat, a cartoon dog, but there is always a pet show. There is always a family. There is always a deep drama, and there might be an offset really intellectual film. But the one that really kicks America is the comedy. You know all of the top movies of the Oscars were playing, but you know which one had three screens? A silly comedy. So we all kind of want entertainment to mean laughter, joy, and levity, right? But in reality, there are sixteen other theater houses, where everyone spreads out to see different movies. So when you are on the table and you see the horror inside . . . it's included in this 99 percent entertainment. Yah? When you see the "puppy movie," it's all inclusive in this 99 percent entertainment.

judgment. Right? That's what I am trying to tell you that you need to reverse a paradigm from. So that the self-trust comes to you, and you do not depend on the receiver to give it to you. This is critical. Why? Because it's you who have the belief systems that have expanded. It's you who has shape-shifted the energy from within you, holding the emotional space. And the receivers can't trust beyond their belief system. So it's up to you.

The other reason is you do know your trust is invested in the support that you get from your light. It's not dependent on them, it's in you. So you need to reverse the self-trust from outer strokes to inner knowing. And trust before you're working on that person. And whatever they are working on, you're not involved for the validation of completion.

You are doing it for yourself. They just so happen to show up. You are happy that they so happen to show up and share that and give you trust. It has to come from you first. You have to reverse that polarity and say, "I trust myself big enough, more enough, that when I am working with that person, they will get what they want to receive, but I am not dependent on them liking me or on them liking the process.

Because if you depended on them liking the process, you can only deal with those who went to the movie about Big Mama's House. You cannot deal with the people who come to the movie about horror, or any of the other of those entertainment forms.

Take a minute. I know that was a big concept, so I say it now. You have to depend on the trust that you have. Before you can turn it over, that power over to someone else. And when you do that, you are always empowered. As soon as you depend on someone else to give you validation, in Lomilomi, it's a wash, that 1 percent will not show up. You will give a massage, and it will be good. But that 1 percent cannot show up, if you don't trust yourself first.

. . . And that's what we are going to work with for the next four days. So that you can feel comfortable and secure and solid. The word is *Pa'a*. So the word in Hawaiian means to be authentic

WITNESSING IS THE HUMAN EXPERIENCE

I tell you, this process of witnessing is the human experience.

OK, I going to say it again.

The process of witnessing is the human experience.

And it does not belong to any dialect of religion. That's what

body workers have to offer: witness. That's a technique.

Not your hands, but your soul hearing. The deeper

you can hear what is going on for your receiver, the more

expansive your capacity to witness it will be.

Then you get into body work. And not necessarily with

your ears—you can also do that with your hands.

But witness is the human experience. Some people will tell you

that relationships are. Again, witness is the human experience.

Relationships are just an extension of that witness.

unto yourself with the weight of your Earth. Your weight to your Earth is so authentic, that you are Paʻa—cannot be moved and swayed by other people's emotion.

QUESTION FROM PARTICIPANT: Do you also mean grounded?

HARRY: Grounded. Perfect word. Paʻa.

If there is any experience I have on the mainland it is that I walk around with Paʻa, and everybody walks around, right here, above the shoulder. So that is what they come for. My sense of trust of myself, that I can sit on the planet, with my feet to the planet, and be grounded to it. That's what draws receivers. Because it stands out! It stands out as something that is connectable. So, Paʻa.

You can take that: "I am Pa'a." And that means that I have enough self-trust to expose to myself, my authenticity. Big one.

Take a breath. "Hu-ah." Take a breath, "Hu-ah."

You will grasp your capacity; you have this capacity to reverse the polarity paradigm of your self-trust. You have that capacity. You have that capacity in the process of "witness." That is what you get to do with each other, and you practice it, and you get it.

7. You will manage energy to three spaces of consciousness: asleep, awake, and aware.

How many people recognize that they are sometimes asleep, sometimes aware, and sometimes awake? One of the things that draws us to body work, is that in body work we can achieve awareness. Yah? Raise your hand if you have achieved awareness during body work, working on someone. Yah? Everybody? Some? That's that 1 percent I am talking about. Does that make sense to you? That's how that fits in.

That's that 1 percent, the awareness. How many believe that they have done body work asleep? I raise my hand first because I know that is true. Right? How many know that though? When it's actually happening?

And then there is awake. Now, awake is that state when you are doing a massage, and you are thinking about not feeding the cat. Right? So it's easier to be asleep and aware than awake. Because awake, you are not even there. Asleep you are there, your body is showing up. And awake, right? "I wish somebody would get that mosquito out of my room." Or, " I wonder what is playing in the theater tonight." That is "awake." Awake is unfocused.

You can shift back and forth. And you have every right to do that. You are human. That's not the experience of holding yourself accountable. You only need 1 percent of God. And that is absolutely life shifting for that person. He is a powerful guy! One zap, and it's over, right?

We are going to cover this concept of Pa'a, the now, several times in this class. Pa'a, the now, is that time before and after what you are thinking. Pa'a, the now, is that time when you have worked so hard and all of a sudden you are on the surfboard and just sailing. Pa'a, the now, is that first bite into the greatest salad that you have ever made yourself. Pa'a, the now, is that 1 percent that you need when you are working with someone. It's when the alignment of your body and your mind and your spirit come into vertical time.

Every kahuna has got to work in the Pa'a, the now. And please, please expand your consciousness to express that *kahuna* in the original language, the encoded language, is not a noun. Take a breath and think about that for a second. *To kahuna* is a verb. It's an activity. A noun is the name of a thing that brings status or "stopping" to something. And the activity of kahuna, which is uncovered light, is a verb. It is a moving stream of intention and intelligence. This whole concept of having a kahuna is not authentic to the language. It is only authentic when it is translated into a culture that has past, present, and future.

Hawaiians did a lot to eliminate that. That is one of the big reasons that nothing is written. Because once it's written, you have past. So *kahuna* is a verb. (*Kahu* and *kupua* are actual nouns, activities that can be labeled. *Kahu* is a teacher. *Kupua* is an architect of belief systems. Big difference!)

Kahuna is an activity that a person participates in, which is to uncover the stream of light. So when you are working with your receiver, that's when you are in the flow of a kahuna. When you are working with your mind in conversation, you are in the flow of a kupua, who shifts belief systems.

It's a verb! Now how does that resonate with you? Does that make sense? Can you make that transition? Because it is critical to go to Pa'a, the now, in this work. We did not record how many moons someone has been. It's not as important as Pa'a, the now.

We try to, the culture tries to, preserve all of its sovereignty to its consciousness. And here is a really important understanding.

I am going to pull this word out, because it really has to do with body work, and the word is *sovereignty*. I know it's expressed nowadays that sovereignty is required for the Hawaiians because they need the land back that was taken. In the kahuna way, sovereignty is not anything about the *Aina* [the land], because no one could actually own the Aina; there was never an argument about that. But sovereignty is the whole reason why Hawaiians will not tell you about this kind of communication, this kind of knowledge. It's because they believe that if you learn Lomilomi and you use technique, you just kind of be quiet inside and listen. You will develop your own sovereignty around the work, because someone will not tell you. Because if someone tells you or shows you a system, you are divorced from creating the Pa'a, the now.

You always have to go back in time to create the system. Does that make sense? Am I making that clear? That is really why. They are trying to empower you by not saying what the secrets are, and

Kupua: Changing Your Belief System

Finally I will tell you, if you find out for yourself, guess who

owns what you know? Aha! And I do that too in this class.

I try to preserve your sovereignty. By not showing you, "This is

where you are supposed to be." Does that make sense to you?

Think about that for a second, it's a big one.

I am not talking about the sovereignty of land rights, I am

talking about the kupua, sovereignty of your being, you

having the ability to grow it, be supported, but not told what

the program is. You will never get to kupua (belief systems) if

you follow a procedure. There is a clear correlation between

your sovereignty and your capacity to witness, your capacity

to hold the grace that comes from God. Does that make sense?

Kupua is belief systems, kapua means flower.

yet they are so misunderstood for doing so. "They always want to keep it secret." No. They are preserving your sovereignty for the connection you need to witness.

That is why I have a huge problem with Continuing Learning Units (the health care equivalent of continuing education credits) and other kinds of systems in teaching this workshop, because they require certain levels of accomplishment and details. "How do we test?" "How can we test this?" You cannot test this. You go in time and are in Pa'a, the now. Nothing else is available to you. Just the grace of God. That makes sense, yah? But it will carry you through any circumstance. There is nothing I have never been able to face on that table—and I face a lot of different hugely complicated circumstances—because I preserve my sovereignty. No one has just told me the next thing to do. So I teach it that way. One tool here and you get a basket with four tools, plus all the tools you already have.

And include them! Because the concept of having 99 percent entertainment with 1 percent God, is 99 percent of you! Brought into the basket so that you can pull it out with the direction of grace. Grace receiving gratitude. Big concept. Grace receiving gratitude.

Thank you for being patient with the language, and I know this is a new language to you, but the concepts will get your body work into the light! With your own sovereignty.

8. *Your unveiled skills will radiate.*

People will feel better, know themselves better, move better, and live better. That will happen. Always does.

So I can sense that everyone's stomachs are a little full, so I am going to ask that you all sit up, take a deep breath. Hu-ah! It's full with poi, heavy, heavy truth.

OK, and I am going to give you a technique, to let it go into your body. To make more sense, it's a really, really simple one, it's a chorus, it's *I'o*. It's a chant, kind of a toning thing. Here we go: I am going to say, "IEO EIO." That's all I am going to say, "IEO EIO."

And for the first time I feel very compelled to tell you what we are saying before we say it. No, I will wait, because it's more intense.

*IEOEIO IEOEIO IEOEIO IEOEIO IEOEIO IEOEIO
IEOEIO* and so on and on.

I'o is the hawk, that Hawaiian hawk that flies highest above
all beings. The hawk is representative of I'o. I'o is a sacred coded
name of the Aloha light. They did not say God for a purpose. The
Hawaiian understanding is once you give God a name, you human-
ize him and restrict his sovereignty. So like the Buddhist tradition
I'o is not the name of God. It is the name of the force that is part of
God. That wind. The *I'o*, the sacred name of God, is never stated,
because it prevents his sovereignty from penetrating to you.

So "IEO EIO" means, in English, grace receiving gratitude.

Now let's look at the definition of grace. Grace is the inalienable right as a human being to receive God's light. That's what
Grace is. Your inalienable right, it cannot be taken away from a
human being.

You can receive God's light, under all conditions in all circumstances. I think that the best way of saying this is, "In God's eyes,
no one is above the other." Yah? "In God's eyes, no one is above
the other." In people's eyes, no form is without God. No form is
without God. So as you are working and you are looking for that 1
percent, you will look for the texture of grace receiving gratitude.
The texture of grace receiving gratitude.

That's enough. I'o is God. You hide the name of God in the
highest flying bird. It's absolutely phenomenal to me that the
Hawaiian culture can close up and leave all these gods visible, and
nobody gets that the gods are simply icons of information. Not
deities below the power of God. That's to take the biggest left turn
that the whole society has made. Ku, Kane, Kaneloa, Lono, or the
four main "gods," are the four schools of thought: engineering,
architectural, farming, and healing. They are not deities or beings
that have creativity power. It's an all-mental experience, too. If you
don't have this all written, you have to have some way to make
icons of the information, to lock into the information. And every
Western person who has come has seen it as a god. But they didn't
understand that god meant "icon of information." It did not mean
the supreme being. So when we talk about coded, let me make it

a little clearer that this is what is coded. It's just CDs, computer code, the old Hawaiian style.

That's all it is. That . . . power of giving came back to them through the concept of "grace receiving gratitude." And it was in check with the light, because it only operated in witness. Yah? Witness. So free is this idea.

I have been accused very often of supporting the Hawaiian culture on the mainland because everybody says: "Hooo, the kahunas were dark." And one of the first things I say up front in the speech when I am hit with that question is, "No, they were not dark, they were deep!" And deep is dark, but not dark that way, in the way that you mean. Dark is from your mind. So because a lot of the reason that they go to this depth is that when you are working on someone, you can not get this idea that all that was explained to you could be actually converted into English.

So you end the session with, "That was ineffable," and they get it. Ineffable, meaning, an idea or activity not conveyable in human language. An idea or activity not conveyable in human language. That's ineffable. That's what Lomilomi gives you at the end of a session, right? So with that we are going to close that, *Pa'u*, that part.

Any questions? I know it's not sitting yet, it's kinda rolling around in there right now, and let that happen.

The Four Declarations

We are going to turn to the next page in your notebook, which is "The Declarations."

If you are wondering why it's not so tightly organized, it's because I want to give you one piece of information at a time. It's hard enough to speak from the now, even though it's printed from the past. I am trying to get it there. Bringing it down to as simple as possible. . . .

The declarations are designed for you to enter into a space of awareness, which is Halau, the comfort zone for learning. And when we have proclaimed them, you have entered into the space to do the work. But they are concepts that you can hold and carry through your work.

1. My presence in the Halau is a sacred manifestation from me to myself, to shower gratitude, growth, and bliss to my whole being.

OK, "My presence in the Halau," that is the presence you have here, "is sacred manifestation from me to myself," so you are giving from me to myself, "showering gratitude, and growth and bliss to my whole being." How many think that they could get that happy? Right?

You got to get that happy when you start a treatment. When I start a treatment I automatically say to myself: "I shower myself with bliss, growth, and gratitude!" I really do. I really say, bliss, growth—sometimes I just hang on bliss, I don't worry about gratitude. I just hang on to bliss, that is all I need. Because I have said this often enough that something happens to trigger my Low Self into the activity. It's going to get excited, a party is coming. You know, it's interesting to notice that in the congress of energy, there is an overwhelming sense of confusion, but if you set a preferred choice, it all flows into a river.

So you are coming into a session, and you have never met this person before, and there is a congress of energy moving through the whole room, and you say "I am here in bliss and joy to shower myself with gratitude, growth, and bliss." And all of a sudden, your power of witness, the energy in the room, all has a flow. All has intent. It knows what to do because you told it! That is what the power of declaration means. So simple, yah? Yeah, it is, because that is how you raise children, you tell them what to do, and they are raised in that source. It's the same thing, you are telling your body what to do in the circumstance. "Be happy!" You have to declare it! Because there are enough forces to say, "Be sad." Especially if no one has said it as one of the declaration's of the Halau (see above). Now, really, you don't have to tell anybody else. You don't have to tell your receiver, "Be happy." You have to tell yourself, "Be happy." Because yourself is where the trust is.

Because if you tell yourself, "Be happy," you have self-trust, it will emanate. You know what *emanate* means? From here, out. "My presence in the Halau is a sacred manifestation from me to myself, to shower gratitude, growth, and bliss to my whole being."

2. I focus to enter into and sustain my temple into Lomilomi, in the pu'u, the heart. That from the heart, through the heart, the essence of my light, my Uhane, supports, guides, and graces my touch.

That's a whole big statement right there, and we are going to chew it up. Because we want you to really understand it. As you prepare to declare it.

"I focus and enter into and sustain my temple into Lomilomi." So in other words there is a temple in Lomilomi that is a space that you can create in your mind. But it always sits in your heart. Now in Hawaiian healing, your heart is where you are working. Both in the ethereal and the spiritual space, as well as the physical space. This is where the Lomilomi temple is, your self-trust. When I say *physical*, I mean aside from other kinds of techniques where you are using your hand and your body. A lot of shiatsu is about working your hips to hold, and to hold that space. If you have ever taken a shiatsu class, it's like that. In Hawaiian healing, you're working from your heart. You're moving the arms and your energy out of the heart at all times. Even if you are moving your legs. Your focus is from the source, your heart. Because the energy that comes from your heart comes also through the Divine from the back of your neck into you, and you never get tired. It's really a stance of holding this space, the heart, open and clear. If you are working from here, the hands, it doesn't work for Lomilomi. It's my experience. I've tried it. It works best from the heart. In other words, if the energy is moving out of your heart and into your hands, your hands don't get tired.

And there's other trick to learn. In Lomilomi, you don't use the hands too much for the rest of the body; you just do some small points in the neck and in the head. The rest is elbow work. So you don't get tired. But that is all to sustain the energy in your body. So you know what I mean—it's about economically using your body.

In an ethereal sense, that is exactly where the energy of grace comes through, your heart energy. Not your mind. The difference between a psychic and an intuitive is that psychics communicate to an entity by their mind. Intuitives communicate to their High Self that speaks to the entity. When you are listening to the language of someone else, if you are hearing it through your heart, it becomes clear that it's a message of intuitiveness.

If it's coming from your brain, it has to process, into future and past tense understandings. Your heart is moving in the Pa'a, the now. That's the big difference. I mean if you just say, "I just know," that's you heart talking, right? If I say "I know because," that's your mind talking. The purpose here is to work through and from your heart. It knows better, we presume that. "From the heart, through the heart, the essence of my light, my Uhane, supports, guides, and graces my touch." Uhane is Spirit. That's what that is. My spirit supports, guides, and grace my touch.

It is critical to understand that your mind is not capable of participating in Lomilomi. Your spirit and your heart entertain your mind in Lomilomi. So you need to free yourself of the "House of Guilt," which is . . . in the mind. Right? Free yourself from that. And trust your spirit and your heart to do the rest.

3. I commit the energy of certainty to the abundance and perfection of my intuition, as I am radiant in the light of Aloha.

"I commit the energy of certainty to the abundance and perfection of my intuition." How many can grasp their mind for a second around the energy of certainty? How many understand how potent that energy is? That it has a different signal from other energies. I am here to nurture with you the energy of certainty in your work. There is an energy of certainty that we can pull out of you. It feels a little parental. Does that make sense? It comes from your High Self. It comes only by invitation. From your mind and your body to your High Self. That's why this piece of declaring it, as we're going to do in a few minutes, brings that attention to you. That energy of certainty.

That is critical in massage. Because you are going to be faced with, like, "Ah! Now I know exactly what to do." Right? You've been there. We're going to make it so that you have the skill to access it at your will. That's what's important. That it becomes a part of your ability to write your name, create the energy of certainty.

It is no coincidence that when you learn Lomilomi in the old traditional style, your life gets really better. Yah? Because you'll have that access to that energy of certainty, which gives you a greater tool. Now it's not all rosey-dosey—there are thorns in roses—but it will be not boring! It will be not boring. Because people on this planet would flock towards the energy of certainty. They always do. They always do. It is the light of God, it should be flocked to. "I commit the energy of certainty to the abundance and perfection of my intuition as I am radiant in the light of Aloha."

OK, I am not sure if everybody knows this story. I always say this at every lecture; it's so important to you. *Aloha* means "the Breath of God is in our presence." The Breath of God is in our presence. In that statement is "hello" and "good-bye" and every-thing else, but you see how it's translated from what we know it as—"hello" and "good-bye," you know?

Football. Everybody in Buffalo says: "Aloha, oh yeah, that football game." Right? Shakes me up. Really shakes me up. So I say at each lecture, *Aloha* means "the Breath of God is in our pres-ence." And that is the radiance that I am talking about.

OK, a last one.

4. "I will my will to compassionate disengagement. And I am sustained by the Breath of God that is in our presence."

So in other words, "compassionate disengagement" and Aloha. Now we really got to get this today, now in the next minute: "compassionate disengagement." One of the things that God does, constantly, is create it, let it go, and observe it, witness it. It, God, doesn't really participate in its completion; it's up to that creation to do that. It sits separate. One of the things we do as parents is, after a certain time, let them make their own process. And disengage from their growth. When you are working with someone, expect them to expand more than you—or not, or not. But be disengaged from their process. If you don't do that, you will not do Lomilomi very long. Most of my experiences in massage school are that 90 percent will take the class and 10 percent will take it maybe two years further. Thirty-six months is the average life of a massage therapist. Thirty-six months. The passion dies. The hurt, the carpal tunnel, all that from the massage practice makes it fall apart. Lomilomi, I think it's safe to say that most people who do Lomilomi do it for life. Because we don't engage in the receivers' drama. Their activity. We have our role. We stay with what's us. We don't project. Whatever is happening to the person in front of you—it's that compassionate disengagement. That's critical to understand. Get that? It's really critical to realize that I am not going to be engaged past the moment of the end of the session. I am not even going to be engaged in the moment of God showing up and their expansion. I am engaged in the activity that generates their sovereign process. You don't want to be taking anybody's sovereignty, right? That's what you do when you engage. Witnessing is not coupling energy. It's reflecting energy. Compassionate disengagement. Huge.

If through the weekend, these concepts will come up and down through your mind, if you need five minutes to really get that point, come and talk to me, because I will find a hundred different ways of explaining it to you. Don't feel that you have to participate in engagement, without that compassionate separation. You can do that. There is a place for that. That is critical to this work. The more you are compassionately disengaged the more grace comes to your receiver. It's just the way it is. I did not design the system. That is the system.

So you can't own them or your work. Have you ever been to someone who owns his or her work? So we know the difference now. It's the polarity/expansion. People who own their work and someone who's free from their work after it is done, right? They can walk away from that completion of the house or the body work, and say, "OK, it's done, move on," versus someone who is, like, hooked into engagement. It's about letting it go, because you have to let it go, because you are in a flow. You are not holding the branch at the side of the river. You are just going with the next thing. It's better. That's why, too, you know. It's really better.

I am going to drop that and ask if anybody's got any questions about those huge things.

Take a minute. Breathe: "Hu-ah." Let it sink in. I feel everybody all full with the stomach with all this food. It's a lot of food that's been presented to you.

Hawaiians really believe energy is food of the being. Now for the last joke: One of the things nice about being Hawaiian is unlike other cultures we don't eat til we're full—we eat 'til we're tired.

And I project that, so I feel you guys look almost tired. That's why I almost stopped talking. But I am going to ask you all to stand—there is no pressure to make a circle—and to make the declarations.

. . . Are we all ready, kinda make a circle so we are all in the same space. We're here to intend to set the space, holding the declarations creating the energy it takes to create the space of the Halau. Which is actually a living intelligent thing, that combination of our energies.

That's what Lomilomi gives you at the end of a session. So we are going to close that, *Pa'u* (finish, end, complete).

Thank you, thank you. *Mahalo, Mahalo.*

Lomilomi Healing Stories

Sue Ann

I first heard of Harry about six months before I met and saw him. An iridologist, Alice Mammoser, I see mentioned there was a man in her building from Hawaii who did body work. I got curious and asked if he would be beneficial for me to see. Her suggestion was see him before I have my next appointment with her. So I did and went about every three weeks for some time, driving the five hours to Buffalo. My medical doctor had diagnosed my condition as a stage four of a rare disease—primary biliary cirrohsis, an autoimmune thing. According to the medical community, there is no cure, but here I am. Now the symptoms are absent.

After meeting Harry and bringing several others to experience Lomilomi, I was very excited to learn that he would be teaching a Lomilomi training class only an hour away from my home. As a registered nurse, I felt comfortable with the concept of Lomilomi and thought I just might be able to offer some of the peace and giving to others that the practice had given me. I choose Lomilomi because I had learned personally to expand and love myself and let it reflect on others who came to me for various reasons.

Harry demonstrated that by entering into helping others to expand you can have deep contact of mind and spirit, and thus both the givers and receivers become stronger, well fed, and expand to become open to possibilities.

Be open to possibilities. Don't be afraid to connect, you will not become lost and submerged in another, but rather find yourself growing and gaining a bit more understanding. The giver and receiver both grow and feed each other.

Trenna

I met Harry Uhane Jim because of something that happened in a workshop over twenty years ago. Before that I thought "the Big Kahuna" was a name made up for the first *Gidget* movie. Afterwards I learned it was the name of a very special person in Hawaii, and my interest in kahuna began.

Since 1983, I have been going to Lily Dale Assembly and have taken well over a hundred workshops. It was during the third summer that I took a class on sacral-cranial work. When it was my turn to receive, I ended up sitting with my eyes closed, in a lotus position on the floor, something I couldn't do before or after that time. (Later I checked again, but I still could not put both feet up on my knees.)

Inside my head, I could hear someone talking, but I couldn't understand the words, they sounded like chanting. I wondered where the sounds were coming from. The urge to express the sounds out loud was strong, but I was reluctant. Finally I could not resist doing it very softly. I kind of hoped no one would hear me. The woman who was working with me told the teacher I was mumbling.

I clearly remember sitting there thinking, "Okay this is a safe place. They won't think I'm crazy. Maybe a little strange, but I could handle that. Besides this doesn't feel like a bad thing." I also had the feeling the teacher would know what I was saying.

Oh well. I took a deep breath and let whatever was inside me come out and express itself as chanting. As the sounds flowed out of my mouth, my hands and arms began to move, they seemed to dance of their own accord in the air. The only clear impression I received about what I was doing was that the sun was somehow important. I felt a peace in my body and rightness to what I was being used to articulate and express.

I still remember the smile on my face as I opened my eyes and so started to see half dozen classmates sitting watching me. They all began to tell me how beautiful what I had been doing had been. I admit to feeling a bit embarrassed by that. You see, I had felt like I was alone in some special place.

Of course I was eager to talk to the teacher to find out what I had said to her.

"I will only tell you this," she said, "I studied in Hawaii and you called me by my secret Hawaiian name. What you told me was a message from my teacher, the kahuna. But that is all I can tell you."

I finally got my wish fulfilled to know more about Hawaii when Harry moved to Buffalo. Harry Uhane Jim, a kahuna, was teaching a class called "Traditional Hawaiian Body Work Medicine Trainings: Enter into the Realm of Lomilomi."

A part of me thought, "This is going to be a great workshop." Another part remembered classes I had thought sounded good turned out be very disappointing. So I was hoping for the best, but I was trying not get too carried away with eagerness.

I didn't see Harry right away when I walked in, because he was tucked behind a corner. When I looked into his eyes, it was as if I was seeing an old friend. And although I very rarely stick my hand out to shake hands, I did to him. He took it. There was a current of connection. I knew Harry was the right person to teach me. This would be a great class, and it was.

So much of what he taught was familiar, Harry puts it this way. "Everything is already known, it simply needs to be unveiled." I agree. I just wish sometimes it were easier to do the unveiling of what I want to remember.

The ten days before Harry's class I had been sick with a lung problem, in need of my oxygen most of the time. I had it on that night so I wouldn't get sleepy. At one point during the class, Harry worked on my breathing. I could feel the energy flow into me as we breathed together. The next day when I checked my oxygen levels they had returned to what is normal for me.

I only needed the extra oxygen at night after that. I was eager to have a private session with Harry doing Lomilomi. I also wanted to learn more.

A few times I had felt Harry's energy when I was meditating. When I asked him about it in the fall, when I went up for a session, he said something like, "When I'm on the treadmill, I open myself to send healing to my receivers."

For about two years I had a recurring flulike problem that made me hurt all over. They kept coming back, and the occurrences were getting closer and closer together. I only go to doctors when I have no other choice. Each time it happened, I did healing on myself and hoped it would be the last. When I started seeing Harry, the episodes were six weeks apart. After working with him four times over a few weeks, and a couple sessions with an acupuncturist, I am doing better. As of this writing it has been five months with not one sign of the "flu" returning.

Harry talked about how Hawaiians teach from mouth to hands. In other words, they tell you about something and you do it. I don't think I will ever prefer a book to a good, authentic teacher like Harry. He offers his knowledge and his heart in the information he shares. Aloha and Mahalo, Harry.

Beverley

In 1995, while in massage school, I read an article about a woman who did Lomilomi on horses. I did a research project on an injured polo horse. I read rudimentary material on Lomilomi, but wished for deeper material. Later I met Harry through a mutual receiver. Lomilomi now provides me with an intuitive stepping-stone towards enlightenment and wholeness—a life flowering. It also provides me with validation for existing knowledge and gives me a thirst for me.

Lomilomi gives permission not to be a slave to structure. Lomilomi expresses the intuitive and nurtures the giver as well as the receiver. It's pure joy.

I am a Reiki master teacher. Reiki, I felt, gave me back the childlike intuitive abilities that society buried. It is difficult to say whether taking Lomilomi before Reiki would have achieved the same results.

I can confidently say that Lomilomi has indeed increased my intuitive sensitivity and brought joy, a sense of nonjudgment, openness, support, love, and comfort. Lomilomi is another step on my path.

Barbara

I have taken Lomilomi training with Harry three times. Also I have been a receiver of Harry's and have a session with him every four to six weeks. Lomilomi makes sense to me. It provides the relaxation of massage and Reiki with the deep penetrating effects of Rolfing. The Lomilomi experience is truly "holistic." It touches every aspect of what a person needs: physically, mentally, and spiritually. Emotionally it interacts with your core and your value systems.

I did not choose Lomilomi; it chose me. I was searching for a greater depth and perception in my life. My path was on hold for a long time. Lomilomi and Harry have opened me up to start again on my path: my search for greater awareness and growth.

The members of the Halau are like a family. Everyone is accepted with love. Everyone respects one another. The Halau expands and grows, but remains personal and intimate. I have copies of the Halau Lomilomi Lapa'au declarations (see chapter three) in my work office. I read them daily, especially when I am having a difficult time—then I am grateful for having met Harry and Sila. I have a "gratitude attack," as Harry would say.

After taking Harry's certification course three times, I had a tearful reunion with my first Rolfer. We had our first meaningful meeting in ten years. We met as equals. That is what the Halau experience has given me—meeting/accepting people as equals with healing gifts exchanged. So many changes have happened to me as a result of the Halau and Harry. Lomilomi has changed my life. I realize now I am not a political game player at work or in business. I'm trying to live my life in a kinder, more loving manner. It's a very hard choice. I am looking forward to the challenge. I always thought of my Lomilomi practice as for the future, for my retirement. Now I realize that I need to put Lomilomi into practice *now*! Not only to benefit my receivers, but for my benefit. "To entertain me," as Harry would say.

Mary

I met Harry about three years ago. Lomilomi provides me with relaxation and helps remove tension and negative energy from my body. I choose Lomilomi because it's much more than a massage. You can actually feel the energy move when Harry's pressing on the pressure points on your body. Then I started taking his classes.

During one of the classes, I attended with a headache that I had all day long. Initially, I was hesitant to go to the class because of the way I felt. Ultimately, I was so glad I made the decision to go. Harry Jim pressed on certain pressure points on my neck, and within minutes my headache was gone. He is a compassionate person, and his practice is quite unique to my local area in general.

Anonymous

I attended a four-day workshop on the recommendation of a friend. Lomilomi helped me get a deeper sense of joyfully releasing that which binds and creates dis-ease in the body. In the healing process, the conduit (giver) and the receiver dance in the movement of energy, one smoothly breathing and dancing with the other. And the Halau presides. Many times, in my Jin Shin Jyutsu practice, I begin with opening up with Lomilomi and ending with Jin Shin Jyutsu—very effective.

Margaret

I am a firm believer that people come into our lives to get us from one place to another. Harry Jim was introduced into my life by a friend and from that moment my journey has become easier.

Together with my friend, I took Harry's "Halau Uhane Lomilomi Lapa'au" classes and training and received a certification in traditional Hawaiian healing. That was two years ago.

I suffer from fibromyalgia (FMS), myofascial pain syndrome (MFP), osteoarthritis, and other physical ailments. I am in pain every day. Harry has treated me for these conditions and relieved some of the pain with Bone Washing. In Bone Washing, the work is best done with the receiver and the giver in thoughtful communication, so that blockages will leave the area in which they are held. Harry, Lomilomi, and the secrets of Aloha have made my life more bearable.

Harry Jim is a very gifted and talented professional. His presence is calming and gentle. He makes me laugh, which in itself is healing and beneficial to my soul and healing process.

Most importantly, Harry and his family have become my friends and gratefully, I continue to learn from them. Aloha!

Sylvie

I did two workshops with Harry at Yoga Oasis in Hawaii. Lomilomi is the best thing I can do for myself. It brings me into a loving state, connecting me with healing power. It certainly benefits me as much as it does my massage receiver.

I was doing water massage for many years and was not attracted to table massage. But the minute I encountered Lomilomi, I knew it was for me. It is much more than massage. It is loving, healing. We work on the body but there is something else happening.

Thank you, Harry, for your great talent as a teacher, to transmit the unspeakable.

Pat

Lomilomi is like communion, where I feel a sense of closeness with God. I always feel pure and privileged when working with a receiver doing Lomilomi. I am a holistic giver, having studied many healing modalities—Reiki, hypnosis, craniosacral, healing touch. I am a seeker and enjoy learning new modalities.

The uniting with breath of life has shown me the path to allow and accept. I am not alone when I am practicing Lomilomi. I have recently worked with three separate receivers, two with right shoulder pain and one with a numb heel. Each person felt great improvement after receiving the Lomilomi treatment. They had tears of gratitude. They truly felt Harry's saying "I am enough."

Anyone can learn and practice if they are of a pure heart and their intention is to heal their Self, heal others, and heal Mother Earth through the Halau. What a gift—to forgive, to let go, to be free and feel God's grace.

Michele

Here is what Lomilomi truly means to me—um, like, *everything!* But to be more specific—I wasn't kidding when I said I needed the weekend intensive like I needed the air. And I'm not kidding when I say that Lomilomi has provided for me access to *everything* that I have been searching for far too long.

When I first heard Harry speak about Lomilomi at Lily Dale in August, it was like coming home. He said so many things that just felt so right—and I wanted to know more. So I booked an appointment with the kahuna and promptly found out just how powerful and life-changing Lomilomi really can be. I can honestly say that things were never the same after that session with Harry, and it was nothing less than truly amazing! (I know that word *amazing* gets overused a lot, but in this case that word was 100 percent accurate.)

That is why attending the workshop in February meant so much to me. That weekend helped me to realize the power in gentleness and the beauty that all of us possess. I learned to appreciate what each of us has to offer one another and the value that comes from being in the moment. I learned that to lead from the heart is truly what is always best in the moment and that is where true power lies. It was beautiful to witness compassion in action throughout the entire weekend.

Being introduced to, becoming aware of, and participating in the Halau over that weekend brought many profound experiences and undeniable connections to a force greater than our individual selves. Feeling the connection to that unconditional support has provided much-needed help in the mending or fixing of my broken heart. I had been searching everywhere in an attempt to regain my emotional balance, to connect to the inner stability, but to no avail. That is until one summer's night, I came across a kahuna on the mainland, far from home, and through him found my way back to my home: my heart. That was the beginning of the beginning, of a new way of life and living.

In short, I feel like I have been living without Aloha most of my life. And this is why I needed Lomilomi like I needed the air— because Lomilomi provided for me the safe place to allow myself to stop and breathe. Working with the kahuna, being able to stop and "take a breath" is enabling me to gain my emotional balance again. And this is priceless to me.

My first session with Harry allowed me to let go of some pretty awful feelings that I just could not get resolution from, no matter how hard I had tried with other methods and philosophies. Lomilomi provided the emotional support that had eluded me most of my life. It is no surprise to learn that *Lomilomi* is actually a verb. And that is why it has had such a profound impact on my life. And because Lomilomi is a verb, it lives—it acts, it grows, and it blossoms. It *provides* emotional comfort and doesn't just talk about it. I have found Lomilomi to be *alive* with life and love. To me, it is thought in action—a loving thought in action, a way of *being* not just thinking. Lomilomi is not just a "positive thought" or feeling. It is full of life, full of emotion, filled with grace, the containment of everything. And this is why Lomilomi has meant everything to me!

William

I choose Lomilomi for clan awareness.

Mary and Family

I met Harry Jim when a friend invited him to Fonthill (a town in Canada). My husband, Paul, and I really liked him. We had lost our son nine years ago, and in the grief lost touch with our daughter-in-law and grandson. My husband was in great pain in his shoulders. I am a former registered nurse, now doing alternative therapies using dark field microscopy with the QXCI/SCIO machine doing live blood analysis, which evaluates and treats with an ion cleanse at the same time. It takes out toxins. The machine is made in Hungary. We escaped from Hungary with twelve families, all of German ancestry, in 1944. My father was German, my mother Slovak. Their families had lived in Hungary for three hundred years. We left in covered wagons pulled by horses, driving our cattle with us for food. I was four. Then we were taken all together to Germany in cattle cars and sprayed with DDT, which is why I got breast cancer at age thirty-one. Eventually eight of the families emigrated to Ontario together. There was a lot of heartache and grief in all our cells.

In Canada, at age fifteen, I worked in the tobacco fields to earn money for college. I have a bachelor's of science in Nursing from the University of Toronto and a master's in Clinical Behavioral Science from McMaster University. Eventually I worked with mentally disabled children after a Canadian Centennial Program identified numerous children not qualified to attend even nursery school. A visiting-nurse service was launched to find and identify these children. Eventually, nine developmental centers were opened as alternatives to schools. I worked there for most of my career. I've spent my life getting people out of institutions across Canada.

Yet with the breast cancer in 1971, I found most of the support groups were pity parties, not focused on advocacy and prevention. I was appalled. It took me a few years to take over the group, but now we are an activist group, raising money for AIDS. I guess you could say I am a crusader/reformer.

Using the QXCI was the closest I could get my husband to relieving his pain over his son's death. For he did not realize that his grief pain registered in his muscles. All of us, my entire family, had pain in the shoulders, all in the same place, like carrying a coffin. I know that if you can heal one generation, you can heal the others, past and future. That day we first saw Harry, my father's spirit came into the treatment room. We have had six generations healed by Lomilomi. I could see the potential—how Lomilomi could help our family. Harry said your own house is a place of healing. That three-cornered tree in the nook of three threes, that's a place to thank the Spirit. Harry was just back from doing a wedding in California, overlooking the Pacific, where a white owl told him to pray and to burn sage on our property.

My mother, who was in a lot of pain from her gall bladder, had two or three treatments with Harry. My mom, who was eighty-five, didn't understand that her shingles were emotionally based. She was listing to one side. After her treatment she went down the walk straight. Her sorrow was her pain. When Harry treated her for her gall bladder, there was no sign of the pain. Afterwards, she did not need an operation. Yet, she went quickly from heart failure not from a gall bladder attack. Harry said she chose not to stay any longer. Harry told us it was OK to let her go. I thought it would be a lot harder to do that, but we were able.

Now I am in good rapport with my daughter-in-law, too. Lomilomi brought her back into the fold. Harry moves toxins out. As with a good Epsom-salts soak, the toxins leave.

The first time I had a Lomilomi treatment I totally went into trance. Into Pa'a, the now, and lost time. The next time, no matter what Harry touched, I cried. The sessions were more than just therapeutic. Our family was healed.

Illona, Mary's Daughter-in-law

My mom [this is what Illona calls Mary] recommended I have a treatment with Harry mainly for a back injury. My C5 and C6 vertebrae were inflamed. My shoulders hurt. I had been working with brain-damaged clients when my left hand was pulled, hard. I had been doing therapies covered by Workman's Comp, yet physical therapy seemed to make it worse.

What Harry does really works. And Harry doesn't do exactly the same thing every time. Not going over the same trigger points over and over. First, he watches me walk down the hall, swinging my arms. He has a keen observation before he ever touches me. He really takes a good look before a treatment.

Illona's Son, Andrew, Age Eleven

My grandma takes me to see Harry because sometimes when I am playing the cello, my shoulders hurt so much. Harry does something to my feet and upper back and neck—so many places—and it is so soothing.

He uses oils and a whole bunch of touching points.

Before, I used to feel so tired, now I am not tired. I feel up. And I can hear the difference in the music because I am not slouching. I have no problem playing for two and half hours. I see other things, too. I see brightness all around Harry.

*　　　*　　　*

Aloha, we have come to the end of our story, dear readers, Aloha nui nui.

Mahalo!

Glossary

We have included this glossary to help you, our dear readers, with a short overview of the mystical Hawaiian terms taught in depth in *Wise Secrets of Aloha*. Remember, Hawaiian words have an amorphous quality. Meanings evolve with variations in tone, sound, context, and the emotional frequency emanating from the breathing of the speaker's body in the moment. Therefore there are layers of meanings in each word. The layers tier from literal to spiritual—all range and blend like the seven colors of the rainbow. The consciousness of the Hawaiian language provides an expanding vessel, carrying thought and the power of thought from one person to the next.

For example, early missionaries put together the word *I'o* as being the noun representing the Hawaiian hawk. But to the Hawaiian kahuna, I'o was the ineffable supreme being whose consciousness cannot be communicated in a noun. The hidden understandings say God is a verb. *I'o* is the verb meaning God. When a Hawaiian kahuna says *God* that term may not be your term, but it still means the holy whole.

Hawaiian words, when the missionaries arrived, were all oral, based on rich, round vowels and rhythm. The missionaries quickly put together dictionaries based on their hearing, their filters, and their projections. So the words were given mostly American

English sounds, which were only approximate. For example, there is a sound in Hawaiian somewhere between the T and the B, but really neither. Try finding that middle sound. Not really possible in English.

The first attempts to communicate Hawaiian esoteric teachings were based on the missionaries' somewhat flawed translations of the Hawaiian language, and therefore the essence of the esoteric teachings wasn't communicated accurately. All ancient, prewritten teachings, such as Buddhist, Christian, Hindu, and native teachings, were infused by divine presence, and then written down by scribes. Papa David Kaonohiokala Bray never wrote down a single teaching; all of his teachings were infused by Presence and then scribed. Auntie Margaret Machado has not written a single teaching; she infused people who scribe. Anyone who writes spiritually will acknowledge that they are inspired. Also, there is in the present evolution of the Hawaiian language that visitors may see on a menu. If you hear the word *Lomilomi*, or any Hawaiian word, diving deeper, snorkeling the Hawaiian language like the ocean, will show you the hidden beauties of the words.

Remember, literal and spiritual meanings. Both are the wise secrets of Hawaiian language.

Aina: Literally, the land. Spiritually, the sentience of sacred Mother Earth, the earth element. The state motto for Hawaii is *U'a mau I ka aina I ka pono*: "the land is perpetuated in its righteousness." To Hawaiians, all land is sacred. These are specially consecrated lands in the Hawaiian islands.

A Ke Akua: "By your power and agreement, I open the port." In the missionary translation of the Hawaiian Bible, this is God the Father of Jesus Christ. Spiritually, the authentic energetic signature of All-Being at the highest frequency of expression.

Ali'i: Hawaiian royalty.

Aloha: "The breath of God is in our presence" (see chapter one). Literally used as a greeting, "hello" or a parting, "good-bye."

Spiritually, *A* or God; plus *Lo*, meaning bridged, infused, connected; plus *Ha*, breath or the activity of breathing, aliveness. A blessing in the declaration of being.

Au'makua: Literally, "the god self of the triune human being." Also your infinite mind or the flame of divine light in you. Spiritually, refers to personal guardians or protectors.

Creating Space: A Lomilomi touch-therapy technique that opens a receiver's clogged energy and makes a channel for the energy to run smoothly throughout the body, mind, and emotions.

Giver: A person giving a Lomilomi session; the practitioner. (See also *Receiver*.)

Ha: Literally, "breath." In Lomilomi treatments, it describes a deliberate process of breathing in through the nose and out of the mouth deeply and completely, making the "ha" sound on the exhale. This breathing is intended to enjoin the presence of the verb of God to heal through emotional evolution.

Halau: Literally, "a meeting house, a place to gather." Also may mean large, numerous, much. Most modern references are to individual schools teaching Hawaiian dance, or hula. Spiritually, Halau is the esoteric field for creating knowledge and a comfort zone where we absorb knowledge. Halau is also a gathering of multidimensional beings who support healing. It is a powerful, amorphous term that expands throughout life as consciousness expands. Its medicine comes from the ancient ways of Hawaiian culture.

Halau Uhane Lomilomi Lapa'au: The name for the esoteric school for creating knowledge of the spirit of healing-touch medicine, founded by kahuna Harry Uhane Jim and Sila Lehua Bray Jim.

Haleakala: Literally, "house of the rising sun." Native Hawaiian esoteric teachings say this is where the planet's ethereal umbilical cord connects to the universe. Also a national park on Maui with a currently inactive volcano.

Hina: Literally, "gray" or "silver." Also, in the circle of Hawaiian deities, Hina is the healing matriarch, an intelligent immortal energy of the feminine. In Hawaii, all islands with high-range rainforests have a blanket of misty clouds enveloping the morning landscape. These clouds are the energy of Hina, in the shape of Auʻmakua, in the lineage of Uhane, bloodline of healers' namesake.

Hina ha Uhane: Literally, "the mist in the mountains." Spiritually, the breath of the healing sister of Pele, who is an immortal being of fire energy and the fire goddess of Kilauea volcano. *Hina* means "sister"; *Uhane* means "spirit of healing."

Hoʻo manamana: Declarative phrase that says everything is a manifestation of divine energy. *Hoʻo* means "to cut through the water," "to move through the water." See also *mana.*

Hoʻopaipai O Ke Nalu: Literally, "to encourage, rouse, stir, excite." In surfing, to call in the perfect wave. Spiritually, it is a proclamation commanding the energy of elements to join your will, to ride from the force of an emotional wave, or commanding your being to use your emotion to ride away from a trance.

Hula: Traditional Hawaiian sacred dance. *Hu* is to work, *La* another code word for Light. "To talk to God" is another way of saying Hula.

Huna: Huna is an ancient Polynesian teaching, holding science-based principles that evoke mastery over the physical plane.

Iʻo: Literally, a Hawaiian hawk who is far-seeing and flies the highest; therefore, Iʻo is omniscient, or all-seeing.

Kahili: "Keeper of the mountain."

Kahuna: 1. According to Papa Bray, Sila's grandfather, known as the Red Hot Kahuna, *kahu* means an honored or high servant/caretaker who has or takes charge of persons or property; *na* means calmness and quiet evolution of the emotions. Thus, a kahuna is the high, calm servant of those who may be seeking higher evolution emotionally. Papa Bray also said kahunas are the shapers and managers of belief systems. (Papa Bray was the first legally recognized kahuna by the state of Hawaii. Others were later recognized through the American Indian Religious Freedom Act of 1978.) 2. Literally, a priest, sorcerer, magician, wizard, minister. Spiritually, an initiated native Hawaiian master who has served apprenticeship, been tested through inner and outer trials, and is acknowledged by the Halau of other Hawaiian kahunas on this and higher planes. Also means "keeper of the wise secrets." An accomplished healer, political advisor, taro master, master of the stars for sea journeys, and so much more.

Kai: Literally, the sea, seawater, "near the sea," "beside the sea." Spiritually, the revered great ocean of life.

Kalaʻe: Clear, calm, unclouded. May also be a personal name.

Kalaʻi: Literally, "to remove debris from taro waterways." Spiritually, the Lomilomi technique of Bone Washing the periosteum by clearing the path of blocked energy so energy flows cleanly.

Kalao: Literally, "the dawn to dawn." Spiritually, enlightenment, to enlighten.

Kaluʻu: Literally, "to sweep and swerve," as a wind gust.

Kane: *Ka* is the root syllable of the Hawaiian triune being of humanness; vibrationally Kane is the congress of our three selves.

Kaonohiokala: Kahuna Papa David Bray's Hawaiian name, meaning "Seeing Eye of the Sun."

Kapu: Set of Laws of the Hawaiian community that prevent passage, or behavior of some kind. The "boundary to be respected."

Kula: An area on Maui.

Kumu: A teacher, as in a hula kumu, a teacher of the sacred dances.

Kumulipu (also *Te Kumulipu*): The Kumulipu is the ancient chant of four thousand generations of the Hawaiian people, which takes three days and three nights of continuous chanting to complete. It records Hawaii's genesis and every clan of the original people.

Kupua: An architect of belief systems.

Lapa'au: The practice of medicine, to treat with medicine, to heal, to cure.

Laulima: Literally, "many hands." Cooperation, joint action, a group of people working together. Spiritually, many hands coming together for healing, to raise the vibration.

Lehua: The red flower blossom from the ohia tree, often strung in leis. (The ohia is the first to seed, grow, and blossom after a lava flow.) It can also be a woman's name, as in Sila Lehua.

Lei: A garland of flowers prepared to raise vibrations. Also bestowed as signs of respect and thanksgiving. Leis are tossed and floated in the ocean in farewells and funerals, and there are special leis for weddings.

Lomilomi: Literally, "to shift." Used to describe a salmon salad with red onions or a masseur, masseuse. Spiritually, vibrational energy–touch therapy.

Lono: A major god concept brought from Kahiki (also known as Tahiti), the god of rain.

Mahalo: Thank you. Gratitude expression. Always used in present tense.

Maka: An eye, "eye of the needle"; the face, countenance; presence; sight, view, lens of camera.

Mana: Supernatural or divine power; life force stored in the triune person's body, mind, and spirit. *Manamana* is *mana* repeated for emphasis. In Huna, mana is represented by water.

Mano: A shark. For spiritual reasons, it is against the law to kill a shark in Hawaii.

Moana: Gaia, Mother Earth as a living, conscious, sentient being.

Nui: Big, large, great, greatest, extremely good.

O'ahu: The most populous Hawaiian island.

Ohana: Family, relatives, kin group, related, extended family, clan.

Pa'a: Literally, firm, solidified, adhering, durable, fast, fired. Spiritually, "the now," as when you standing on a surfboard with all your attention focused on the moment and you are one with the elements.

Pele: lava flow, volcano, eruption, volcanic activity; named for the fiery volcano goddess, Pele.

Poi: A staple food in Hawaii.

Pono: Rightful, righteous, or in balance.

Pu'ka: Shell. A type of shell that has a hole in the center making it very easy to string together.

Pu'le: Literally, prayer, blessing, grace. Spiritually, understanding the laws of manifestation.

Puna: An area on the big island of Hawaii.

Pu'u wai: Literally, "A spring from which water comes out." The source of a river. In creatures the heart from which the blood flows. Spiritually, the energetic heart.

Receiver: A person receiving the healing in a Lomilomi session; the client or patient. (See also giver.)

Temple Lomilomi: Body work raised to the level of spiritual healing.

Uhane: Spiritually, "the conscious Spirit of Will"; a person's emotionally mature voice. More like *buddhi*, the wise mind in Buddhism, than *ego*, the psychological term.

Unihipili: The Low Self—the third self of the triune being. The consciousness of the body and the unconscious mind.

Unconditionally loyal and extremely moral in character. Without voice, the Unihipili is subservient to ego and a willing servant and recipient of Spirit.

Wai: Fresh water or any kind of liquid other than seawater.

Waialeale: The name of a mountain on the island of Kauai.

Wailua: The name of a river in Kauai. Also means a spirit, ghost, remains of the dead.